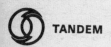
TANDEM

The New Childhood

How does one become a 'good' parent? The New
Childhood, which offers answers to questions like,
'Who is to be boss in your house—your child or
you?' or 'How can I stop him from . . .?', helps
you to prevent the situations which create problems
of parenthood you can't handle. Erna Wright
doesn't say, 'You ought to do this, or that'; instead
she shows ways of handling life with your under-five-
year-old which are based on her own experience.

She writes as a mother and grandmother, not for
the theorists and the experts, but for other mothers,
aunts and grandmothers—and fathers, uncles and
grandfathers—and she has a refreshingly no-
nonsense, practice-rather-than-theory approach to
life with an under-five-year-old.

Also by Erna Wright

THE NEW CHILDBIRTH   Tandem edition 30p

The New Childhood

Erna Wright

TANDEM
14 Gloucester Road, London SW7

First published in Great Britain by Allan Wingate
(Publishers) Ltd, 1972
Published by Universal-Tandem Publishing Co. Ltd, 1972

For Lara
(we laugh together and I am her Grandmother)
and all her contemporaries,
in them our fondest hopes reside.

Hampstead—London—Springtime—1971

Printed in Great Britain by litho on smooth wove paper
by Anchor Press, and bound by Wm. Brendon,
both of Tiptree, Essex

Contents

Introduction

I SUSPECT that you are reading this introduction because you are already a parent or because you are expecting to become parents soon. So it's too late to debate about having a child. The die is cast; you have joined the club; you are one of us. You will spend the rest of your life needing to be a teacher, a guide, a nurse, a companion, an absolute authority, a symbol of the roots every human being puts down in some way in some place—a parent.

Loving your child is instinctive; liking him or her is something else again. It presupposes he or she is likeable—and to turn a demanding, selfish newborn baby into a nice, biddable five-year-old takes a hard slog we call upbringing. That's what *The New Childhood* is about.

Now I know this isn't the first book on the subject. There's at least one every decade, written according to the current wave of thinking. There is nothing which changes as fast as fashion—in clothes, pop music, films and, odd to say, in the handling of the job of being parents. Volumes could be recorded about instances of difference between the dogmatic approach to every aspect of a child's routine laid down only thirty-five years ago and the totally permissive attitude sometimes advocated now. *The New Childhood* is not fashion-conscious. After all, babies are humans, and they don't alter all that much over the years. There are bound to be certain basic theories which work, even though they might appear in a new form.

True, each individual grows and changes all the time, but

the path of change follows certain landmarks. This book—
gleaned from my training as a nurse, my experience as a
mother and my observation of miniature mankind in general
—is an attempt to help parents recognise those stages and steer
through the maze of prejudice and advice, both good and bad,
which they'll doubtless meet once they find themselves with a
son or daughter.

Son or daughter, him or her . . . Can we agree right now
that I shall refer to your child as 'him'; but even if 'he' is a little
girl, rest assured it is still your child I'm talking about. Most of
the time, that is . . .

I can't guarantee that *all* children will behave alike in similar circumstances, of course. They're not puppets, thank
heaven, who all react in a certain way because we pull certain
strings. I can only generalise. So every time your infant be-
haves in some inexplicable way which does not conform to
what my book says, just take comfort from a fellow sufferer. I
have three highly individualistic children, none of whom did
precisely what the pamphlet I was using insisted they'd do!
The point is to learn to cope with your own child's nature, and
that's what I hope to show you how to do.

Cope . . . perhaps that word conjures up the wrong image.
It sounds rather as if we're looking at the picture of parenthood as an ordeal, seeing only the crises and the tantrums and
the colic and the hormone-infested teenager who does not know
if he is an adult yet.

So let's think about the rewards instead. Now if you expect
to feel any sense of reward right from the word go, perhaps
when you come home from hospital, you are doomed to disappointment because your sense of how exciting, how wonderful, is liable to be clouded by all the things you feel you are so
inexpert at, so *bad* at. Then suddenly one day you find that
something or other you've done for your baby—you've fed
him; you've changed him; you've put him back in his cot:
whatever it is—doesn't seem to be so bad, because at least you
haven't caused havoc; your child isn't resisting or furious or
upset. Quite the contrary: he's silent, and later on perhaps he's
even smiling at you. And you think: 'Yippee!' This is the
first sign of reward.

Now the sense of being rewarded goes on during your relationship with each other, even when the child is no longer a child but somebody else's husband or wife. But it tends sometimes to be overshadowed by anxiety, irritation or fear, and on these occasions you wonder: 'God, was it worth becoming a parent?'

But I'm sure that the times when you feel how nice it is, what fun, easily outweigh the others—providing you are reasonably intelligent about your function as a parent. Even so, I feel it's important to point out that it is not a crime, it is not a sin, you are not an unnatural parent if once in a while you are driven to say: 'Oh, I wish I hadn't!'

Being intelligent parents means using your common sense, your instinct, and being selective about the advice you get from well-meaning friends, or for that matter from professional experts, or even from me! It means learning to live as a family instead of as just a couple. Equally, your child must learn to live with you. This has perhaps been forgotten by a generation of parents who heard a great deal about the danger of giving children complexes or frustrating them; and so they reared their offspring to think the house ran exclusively for their benefit.

In my opinion this is a bad way to carry on. Every child must learn to fit into a particular household with particular rules and with things which are peculiar to it, just as babies learn to eat the particular national dishes of the countries they happen to be born in. Indian children are weaned on to curry; they go from milk to curry in one jump because that's all there is. And they seem to be doing very nicely, thank you. As long as a diet contains vitamins and minerals and protein, and so on, it doesn't matter much whether it's curry, or ragout or steak and onions. That's what I mean about learning to live in a particular environment.

It is wrong to try to organise one's entire way of life merely to suit one new human being: because whereas a mother might be willing—let us even assume that her husband, under the mistaken impression that this is what fathers ought to do, might be willing—sooner or later there'll be someone in his life who won't be at all willing; and what a rude shock that would be. For instance, if this procedure were repeated when the second baby came, the older brother or sister might well object to being completely reorganised to suit the newcomer. Besides, if the baby doesn't learn how to fit himself into one household, what chance does he have to fit into the world?

We have to be aware all the time that we are not just looking after a baby. We are educating a human being, who must eventually know everything we know—plus, we hope, a little more. This means learning how to survive—being aware of the danger of scissors, electric plugs, saucepan handles, matches . . . It means learning to be socially acceptable— having respect for other people's feelings and property. It means learning self-discipline. Inevitably, this final process starts by learning Mummy and Daddy's discipline.

I know it's hard to disappoint your child and say 'no', but sometimes you must. I've been told about a child who goes to bed every night in wellington boots—yes, honestly. I gather that when undressed after a tiring day outside, the little boy suddenly refused to have his boots taken off. Instead of ignoring his 'Shan't!' and calmly removing them anyway, the intimidated mother faltered, the child shouted louder, and lo and behold this incredible habit was begun. Now apart from the overt harm to his feet and to the sheets, what about the less apparent harm to the boy's character? Moreover, if his parents couldn't make a stand over such a clear-cut question as this, how many other things—perhaps more serious—does he get his own way on?

Now please don't get the idea from this that I regard you as Big White Chief. I don't. You are not the boss; nor is your child the boss. But ultimately, because you are older and wiser, because you have responsibility for him morally, ethically, as well as in law, what you say goes.

Even so, you must be certain that what you say is absolutely reasonable—like 'Now you don't wear your wellingtons to bed; they're ready for the morning when you go out to play again' —and not just a decision you make in a flash of temper, or on a whim to please somebody whose pleasure isn't that important anyway. I'm thinking here of a patronising schoolfriend you wish to impress, or a strong-willed relative like Grandma.

Grandmothers often wield an unholy power over their grand-children, insisting this or that is what should be done. Remember: grandparents had their day with you or your husband; it's your turn now. Be courageous enough to stick to your own beliefs.

Children have a great sense of justice. If you suddenly change the rules to suit an outsider, they'll know it and feel betrayed. Don't you remember how you felt when your boss denied having given you an hour off to have your hair done just because *his* boss was there when you got back?

Generally speaking, your child reacts as you do. Just because he is smaller than you doesn't mean he's of a different species. He will be as hurt by a preoccupied 'Very nice, dear', when he's telling you about a game he's invented, as you are by a 'Yes, dear,' from your husband when he hasn't listened to a word you've said! Your child will be as delighted with a spontaneous hug from you as you will be with a sudden hug from him.

Try to treat him as a *person*, not as something called a baby or a toddler. For instance, if you tiptoe past his pram hoping he's asleep only to discover he's wide awake, say 'Hi' or something. After all, when a neighbour catches you in the garden and mentions the sun's come out, I assume you don't go shuffling on with your head down, pretending to be invisible. See what I mean?

And while we're on this subject, beware of thinking of him as MY child. Certainly you gave birth to him; you provide his comforts; you're his lifeline—but all this still doesn't make him your property. You don't own him; you're only entrusted with his life until he's fit to take over for himself. Yet the concept of 'my child' may suggest to him that you do own him. And it goes both ways: if he's YOUR child, then you're HIS MOTHER.

There are many small children—and it's easily seen in the street, in restaurants, and on trains and buses—who really think they do own their mothers. They command constant attention, and that's not good for either the child or the parent. So encourage your child's independence and hold on to your own. Apart from anything else, the day will come—long after

this book has immediate application—when he will require
something other than the mother-child relationship, and you
have to have that something else available.

Talking of independence, I think perhaps it is important to
mention that, exciting as it is to be a mother, many women
tend to forget this is only a part of their life. To submerge one's
personality so completely that all there is is this symbol of help-
fulness and authority which is motherhood is wrong. One
should make efforts to remain a person in one's own right,
with views and opinions about things other than how to look
after a baby. And one also has to remember one has another
role—the role of wife.

Many difficulties in marriage, many father-child relationship difficulties, occur because unconsciously Father resents the
fact that he has gained a child but lost his wife. It's as though
some women can't be two things to two men at the same time,
even though one of the men happens to be a little girl lying
in a pram. This is why I've always suggested to young
expectant parents that social life doesn't have to stop at this
juncture. And since pregnancy lasts only nine months but
rearing the child takes eighteen years, it's even more vital now
that you keep your social diary going.

You should still keep up with friends; you should still have
a personal life within yourself separate from your relationship
with a child. Presumably you didn't interiorise into your
married relationship so completely that you were no longer a
person in your own right but merely somebody's wife; so in
your new maternal role, don't let yourself become merely somebody's mother. Nature may have intended this; but you're not
a wild animal. Fight the temptation.

Apart from it being better for yourself and your husband
that you should remain Ann or Mary as well as being Mummy,
it's also better for the child. Just imagine how dull it would
be living with someone who can never be a companion because all she thinks about is cooking and bath-nights and
school reports !

This recognition of your right to be an individual is a good
thing which has come in this post-war era. One of the not-so-
good things is a curious desire to find deep-seated psychological

motivations for every response we get from our children. I've seen a little girl fall and graze her knee and shed mighty tears out of all proportion to her injury. Her 'modern' parents then psycho-analysed the situation, deciding that this display of emotion was a subconscious act to frighten them because she felt they rejected her last week. Well, could be . . . But isn't it far more likely that she cried so much because the pain was just that bit greater than she'd experienced before, or because she was tired as well as having this nasty sore knee, and the combination was at that moment unbearable? Don't let a happy parent-child relationship become a treatment. It will only worry you and make the child fraught and unnatural. It is only when a child is obviously seriously psychologically disturbed that a mother needs to be on constant guard, with the guidance of a specialist.

By now you will have gathered that *The New Childhood* is about the How of Childhood, rather than the What of Childhood. It is not intended to be a factual handbook. I won't attempt to deal with all the varieties of patent baby foods, and the advantages of one over another. Nor shall I give precise instructions on nursing a child suffering from measles. Firstly, when your child has measles the person to consult is your doctor; and secondly there are plenty of leaflets, pamphlets, and indeed textbooks very cheaply available which will supply this sort of information. (Incidentally, as we go along through the chapters I may have to mention specific things—a particular piece of equipment or a particular method of sterilising. The ones I name are merely examples and there is no implication that any other brand isn't just as good.)

All very well, you say, but I still want to use *The New Childhood* as a reference book. How do I do it? In the first place there's an alphabetical index at the back; so if you want to find out about transferring your child to a bed from his dropside cot, simply look up 'COT' and read the appointed page.

Alternatively, you can see from the contents page that we've got chapter headings, and Chapter Two, '. . . NEXT TO GODLINESS' is obviously going to talk about washing, bathing, toilet training and so on. Moreover, I've taken the chapters chronologically from 0 to 5 years and, where useful, I've marked the actual age-group I'm discussing in the following paragraphs.

You have, let us say, a nine-months-old baby and every time you attempt to put him on the pot he goes tense, he screams, he kicks; and you achieve very little by way of pot-training. What are you doing wrong? Well, you turn to Chapter Two and you will find toilet training for a nine-months-old dealt with or at least mentioned. Or if you are having difficulty with breast-feeding, you turn the page to Chapter One and find there, we hope, some helpful advice. In fact, why don't we start right now with feeding? I'm calling it 'The Way To a Child's Heart . . .'

CHAPTER ONE

The Way to a Child's Heart
is Through his Stomach

THIS CHAPTER on feeding is going to be one of the exceptions to my rule: it will give certain ideas on *what* to do as well as how to do it. I've decided on this because there appear to be far too many conflicting and sometimes positively harmful views which people follow on the subject; and since feeding a baby forms the basis of his physical and mental growth I think it's too important to leave to chance. So I'm about to hand on some clear, common-sense suggestions about the best method —and I freely confess that the best method is not necessarily the easiest method . . . easiest for Mother, that is.

0 – 3 months

Perhaps the first thing to say is that babies are all individuals. Nobody has a built-in alarm clock. And whilst clock-feeding is virtually essential in hospital because without a routine our understaffed maternity departments couldn't function, each baby in those wards would probably prefer a different meal-time. So as soon as you get your baby home, I think it helps enormously if you allow him to some extent to govern when he eats—and when he eats should be when he's hungry, not when the clock says it's feeding-time. Of course, this *does* work out to five meals in every twenty-four hours, at least in the first three months, but whether some meals have intervals of three hours and others have intervals of seven doesn't matter a scrap.

There is also the controversy about breast-feeding, which perhaps deserves a word or two. May I say breast-feeding is still the finest method of feeding a new baby and giving it a good

15

start in life. But every woman cannot breast-feed. Every woman doesn't want to breast-feed. (In spite of the fact that she intellectually knows the advantages, for emotional reasons we don't need to go into she can't bring herself to do so.)

For both these groups of women, there are good substitutes —substitutes which ultimately will make little difference to the child's development. Of course the immunities and antibodies which the baby absorbs from his mother's milk cannot be put into a formula, but other factors compensate. You must, however, understand that one of the essential differences between mother's milk and most packaged formulae is the sugar content. The intestines of a baby under three months cannot absorb sugar adequately, and therefore many digestive disturbances —the much-dreaded three-months colic, for instance—are often aggravated by the baby's being fed on some milk formula which had sugar added as part of the making up process. There is also the danger that the baby will develop what is known as a 'sweet tooth'—wanting more and more sweet substances as he grows up until he has signed his own warrant for the dentist's chair.

You don't need to court these teeth problems There is at least one milk formula which does not need the addition of sugar—in fact the makers specifically advise against it—and this is S.M.A. Admittedly, S.M.A. is somewhat more expensive than its competitors, but even the makers say that you needn't use it after the first three months, when you can start your baby on ordinary pasteurised cow's milk.

Before we leave the topic of breast- or bottle-feeding, I'd like to talk about that army of women in the middle. They want to breast-feed but find they don't produce enough milk to do so exclusively. In hospital they were probably issued with a 'top-up' bottle, say of about 3 ozs, to give their baby after the breast-feed. Fine then, when there was somebody else to bring it to them.

But if you belong in this category, you will know it's not so good when you get home. There, more than likely, there's just you. And under those circumstances topping-up is the worst of both worlds. You have the longer time-factor (the traditional ten-minutes a side) and the inconvenience of getting undressed and breast-feeding, without the smug consolation that at least you didn't have to pad down to the cold kitchen and mess about with bottles. And in my experience it's the breast-feeding that goes by the board.

This is a terrible shame. So if you can't breast-feed all the time and grow exhausted with the palaver of topping-up, far better to do alternate feeds : for example, a nice leisurely breast-feed around 2 p.m. when there's just you and the baby, and a bottle feed at 6 p.m. when you're also coping with your husband's dinner.

When you should add solid foods is very much a question of what your baby needs. Some babies need solids from as early as three weeks old. One famous London hospital did some research recently where they fed babies solid food from birth, and although there were no particular significant improvements in the babies' development, it certainly didn't do them any harm. But most health visitors and clinic doctors advise that a baby be given just his milk—breast milk or milk formula—until he is obviously no longer satisfied with it and needs something additional.

Then one of the cereal foods—like Farex or Farley's Rusks —can be given in milk in very small quantities. (May I say here use a *plastic* spoon, not Aunt Emily's solid silver christening spoon which will turn black when sterilised in Milton.) Remember that your baby is accustomed to sucking, and the physical action of sucking from a teat or nipple is quite different from taking food from a spoon. Therefore your baby's first attempts at eating are liable to be clumsy. He may well reject the strange method. Persist gently. If you put a crumb on his lower lip, causing him to lick it, he may find the experience so pleasant he's willing to learn to live with a thing called a spoon.

On the other hand it may be the food itself he distrusts. Don't force him on the occasion when he refuses; just give him his milk and try again at the next feed. If his resistance is really marked, leave him for a couple of days longer without his solid food and then try again. It's probably a matter of gradually getting him used to this new sort of taste going into his mouth.

Incidentally, for the same reasons as before, don't add sugar or any other sweetening to cereal. In any case cereal is adequately flavoured to a baby's liking.

In the first three months the addition of cereal is enough for the needs of most babies; so unless the doctor or health visitor suggests that a wider variety of mixed semi-solids ought to be introduced, I should leave it at that. They will also advise you when to begin cod-liver oil or substitute, and Vitamin C. And at the mention of Vitamin C, here I go again. In Britain we are accustomed to using orange-juice or rosehip syrup for this purpose, but most commercially produced juices and syrups contain large quantities of sugar.

Now it does seem daft, doesn't it, studiously to have avoided giving your child his milk and cereal without added sugar, only to undo this good with his fruit-juice? Moreover, it's possible he will refuse to take the cereal or the milk which *doesn't* contain sugar because he craves the sweetness he met in the syrup. So instead buy those cheap juicy Spanish oranges and squeeze half of one a day, giving him the juice to drink. This is admittedly a lot more trouble and a little more expensive than spooning out the commercially-produced version, but if you have your child's health—and here we are talking mainly about dental health—at heart, you will give it a try.

Suppose you are reading this book when your child is already a few months old and you are muttering: 'Heavens, I have given my child sugar, sugar, sugar; sugar all the time. Now I will stop.' Well, you can do, but you'll find you'll have a very unhappy child on your hands for several weeks, and you may well give in in the end out of sheer desperation. So it might be wiser to start by simply reducing the quantity. Perhaps you could also stop using white sugar and use honey or brown sugar as a sweetening agent, or even glucose. But don't assume you can withdraw all the sugar in one gulp, reasoning that because it's good for him he's going to like it. He's not. He doesn't know how painful a decaying tooth can be; he knows only that he's been deprived of his cherished sugar.

It has long been recognised by experts that one of the most important things for a new baby to learn is how to form relationships with the people around him, and for several months to come the biggest opportunity for this is while he is being fed.

Now when a baby is being breast-fed it is almost inevitable that he will be closely cuddled by his mother, but unfortunately it is not automatic when he's being *bottle*-fed. Theoretically one doesn't have to hold him close to the body to get the milk into his mouth; in fact one doesn't have to hold him at all. It is only too possible to leave him lying in his cot with the bottle propped up so that the teat is in his mouth. May I stress here that a large number of babies under the age of six months choke to death every year by being fed in this way. But almost as important as the danger factor is the point that he is being denied the human contact he desperately needs.

It's not really very strange when you think about it. Imagine putting your husband's dinner in front of him every evening and then going off to do something else, so that you never shared the actual occasion of eating with him. Wouldn't he soon begin to suspect your love for him? In our society we use the occasion of eating as an opportunity of strengthening our relationships. That's why we go out to dinner with friends. This is why your husband might take you out to a meal on your birthday : he's using the meal as a means of letting you know that he's fond of you.

For a baby, you can't tell him in words so that he understands it clearly, but you can tell him by the closeness of physical contact. After all, he's had it for nine months. You can't get much closer than living inside a woman's body, and to expect your baby now to be totally independent of you is a little unfair. Besides, for the rest of his life if he's functioning normally as a human being, he will desire to have physical contact with whomever he forms deep relationships. Everything from kissing and embracing to actual love-making are aspects of this need.

In passing I mentioned sterilising equipment for the baby. A word about this. Patricia, who edited this book and is also a young mother, confessed to me that she religiously rinsed round mixing jug, bottles and cereal bowl with boiling water in the fond belief that this killed bacteria. So let me tell her and any other offenders that this rigmarole does nothing but cleanse. Certainly one *can* sterilise with boiling water, but it takes ideal clinical conditions : a container with a tight-fitting lid, boiling for at least twenty minutes, and even then one would have to examine the container, the water and what you do with the bottle after you have taken it off the gas before one could say definitely it's sterile.

It is much simpler and much more hygienic to sterilise bottles, teats, their covers, the plastic spoon you use for mixing milk or indeed for the feeding itself in a solution like the proprietary Milton. If you buy Milton and the little trough which goes with it, you get precise instructions on how to use it to ensure that your baby always has milk out of a bottle which at least started out sterile. Oh yes . . . and if you drop the teat on the floor, don't pick it up and use it simply because it's just come out of the Milton solution. Take it away; wash it later, use another teat from the solution.

As your baby gets to six months or more, there is less and less need to sterilise anything except if he continues to use the bottle and teat for milk. Milk harbours bacteria which are harmful to human beings very easily, and to a young baby gastro-enteritis can be fatal.

For cups and spoons and his bowls and plates, normal domestic washing up will do, not in the greasy washing-up water following the saucepans, but washed first and preferably allowed to dry on a rack instead of being wiped with a tea-towel of dubious cleanliness.

If you have occasion to go out for the day, do take enough bottles with you to give your baby as many feeds as he is likely to need. Bear in mind that you're the one with the Milton. British Railways, your mother, the Townswomen's Guild don't provide it.

3 – 6 months

Now some babies are quite happy on just cereal and milk until they're four or five months old. They're gaining weight satisfactorily; they're bright; they're happy; they sleep well. And until this state of affairs alters or until your doctor or clinic instructs you to do otherwise, you don't have to introduce any new foods. But for the majority of babies, as they pass three months, they'll start to require additional protein and vitamins. So now is the time to show them that not every food tastes like milk.

By the time you read this book you will be aware that there are many tins, jars and packets of food which are sold expressly for babies—baby dinners, baby desserts, baby snacks. (The packets contain dehydrated food, to which you add water, or milk, as required.) I know how convenient a method of feeding a baby this is. Instead of having to play around with little spoonfuls of this and that, having to cook just two small carrots, you simply take powder or a couple of scoops and put the rest back into the cupboard or refrigerator. I know it's easy; I know you have a lot to do; I know that your double role of mother as well as wife probably cuts into your time much more than you realised. Nevertheless, I have to say what I honestly feel : and that is that these foods are all very well for people who absolutely can't help themselves—for people who are on holiday, for people who because of business reasons travel a lot, for people who have to leave their baby with a minder.

But for the average mother, using fresh lightly cooked foods which she herself makes into purée suitable for her baby is infinitely preferable. For instance, there's ready-made lamb stew with vegetables on the market. Well, that's fine. Baby should have lamb stew with vegetables, but he's better off with your version of it. You can control how little (if any) flour your own stew contains. Cornflour is starch, and too much starch means a fat baby. And a fat baby, it has been proved, often grows into an overweight child.

So use your own stock—the butcher will sell you for a very few pennies, and may even give you, bones which you can stew. Add puréed vegetables to that stock and the juice from your own meat, like your Sunday joint. You can also include in his diet the soft-boiled yolk of an egg (the white tends to be indigestible for the first nine months of a baby's life), steamed fish flaked (use a fresh fillet like cod and not something like plaice which has many small bones that you may not be able to see), or grated cheese, which when melted in milk and poured over a vegetable purée makes an excellent substitute for a meat dish. Much the same applies for dessert : give your baby puréed lightly cooked apple, mashed pear or banana, puréed orange, and any of the soft stoned fruits as they come into season.

As a final word on this subject, may I say that if you must use jars, tins, and packets, don't use them exclusively. Add puréed vegetables to his Beef Dinner; stir grated cheese or egg-yolk into his High Protein Cereal whenever you find you can spare the extra preparation time. For making purée buy a Baby-Mouli in any hardware shop.

During this period you will find increasingly that your baby will want to join in the process of feeding. After all, you can't expect him to lie there as he did when he was new, just sucking at the teat or nipple with eyes blissfully closed; now his hand will join yours. If that's all that happens and he remains fairly passive, conveniently opening his mouth at regular intervals like a young bird, jolly good. But you will probably find that his little hand gets in the way; so give it something to do. Many babies are satisfied if you pass them a spare spoon which they can wave in the air while you're using the working spoon.

Other babies are not so easily put off. They insist on gripping your spoon regardless, and you need both your hands to get that banana into his mouth instead of on you, the floor and his chin. If you have one of these determined tough-guys, I suggest you sit him in his Baby Sitta or prop him up in a corner of the couch for his food, cuddling him on your lap only for his milk drink. Even so, he'll probably still attempt to join in by grasping at your hand, your face, the spoon.

All right—it takes longer; it's messier; *you* may have to wear a large apron. But even though your baby's 'help' makes life a little more difficult, try not to discourage it. Unless today is a day when you've a train to catch or Great-aunt Agatha is coming to tea and you want the baby spotlessly clean, let him begin to learn to hold something in his hand and lead it to his mouth. One day soon he'll be able to do so firmly, and this is an exciting step forward.

6 – 9 months

For a variety of reasons, if you are still breast-feeding by the time your baby is six months, I believe you should now start weaning him on cow's milk. You've done a good job, but there's no need to continue. He's had all the vital antibodies from you that he needs, and to carry on breast-feeding regardless is sheer indulgence—either for your baby or for yourself. So start replacing the 10 a.m. breast feed with a bottle, and after about a week—when he's happily adjusted to that change —replace a second feed. If he's still having a 10 p.m. feed, choose that one; if not, make it the 6 p.m. feed. After a further week, replace the 6 a.m. feed. And a week later still, replace the 2 p.m. feed; this should complete the change-over for most babies. But for those who are still having five feeds a day, it will take a final week to cut out the 6 p.m. feed.

I make it all sound very easy, don't I? And fortunately for most mothers it is. But for some it can be uncomfortable, and for a very few, painful. If you're one of the unlucky ones, do go and see your doctor; he can help.

How do you prepare cow's milk for your baby? Measure the right amount of pasteurised milk into his sterilised bottle (see page 20) and stand it in a jug of very hot water to warm to the temperature he likes it. But beware the drips from the outside of the bottle splashing your baby. They are hot!

Babies vary in the length of time they need to drink from a bottle. If your child is content with the bottle and makes no attempt even to reach for a cup, then let him keep his bottle. I have known a number of babies who grew into happy, healthy human beings who, when they were eighteen months old, were eating neatly and tidily with a spoon but still liked to drink— milk, fruit-juice or water—out of a bottle with a teat. Remember, sucking itself is a powerful stimulus which babies need for varying lengths of time. Don't try to make your child grow up before he's ready.

While we're talking about drinking, let me say something about babies' mugs and cups . . . Never, obviously, give your child a glass tumbler; this could be dangerous for him. And I wouldn't give him a china coffee mug either; this could be dangerous for your coffee mugs! The best solution is a plastic beaker or an unbreakable mug. You'll also find on sale plastic mugs that have lids with holes—a sort of half-way house between a bottle and a cup. (Mothercare do a good one.) Six-

and seven-month-olds often take very happily to these, but don't be surprised if your child proves an exception. None of my three children liked them, either; yet they accepted an ordinary beaker fairly readily.

Equally don't give your child a spoon and insist he learns to feed himself. If he wants to, splendid. By now, anyway, he will probably hold a rusk or a piece of toast and suck or chew at it. This is good for his teeth and gums, and good for his learning how to get food from hand to mouth. Certainly he'll never conquer this complex skill if it's only your sure hand which travels the journey. But watch your child. Let this business of feeding himself come about because he, and not you, desires it.

What to feed him . . . Here the process is mainly cutting down the quantity of milk and increasing the amount of solids, until milk becomes a drink rather than his main food. His digestion's getting stronger all the time. Unless food is very highly-seasoned and obviously unsuitable for him, try giving him a little of whatever you're eating. Naturally, mince or purée it to suit him, and he'll probably welcome the variety.

At the end of this period you should aim for three meals a day—a recognisable breakfast, dinner and high tea routine, with water or fruit-juice with his midday meal and the milk he misses as a mid-morning or last-thing-at-night drink. Incidentally, even though your baby may be taking his milk from a cup very happily at all other feeds, you might find he'll want to suck from a bottle for this final one before settling down for the night. As I've said before : he finds the sensation of sucking soothing. Don't deprive him of it without his consent.

How does he give his consent? By not bothering to suck properly through the teat for about three days in succession, but accepting that same milk if you pour it into his beaker. You know then that he's come to the conclusion the pleasure he gets out of his bottle just ain't worth the effort !

And by the end of this period his milk intake should be down to between a pint and a pint-and-a-half per day (ask your health visitor for individual guidance) and that 'snack' feed may well have been cut out altogether.

During the whole weaning period, you need to be sure that

your child's digestive system is dealing with all the new substances. *Watch his stools.* If he becomes constipated or his
motions become loose, eliminate from his diet whatever new
food substance you have introduced in the last twenty-four
hours. Wait for several months before offering that food again.

The other signal to look out for is a rash—not necessarily
all over his body. If this occurs, go to your doctor immediately.
You don't know, but *he* does, whether this is measles or an
allergy to something your child has eaten.

9 – 18 months:

Once your child has several of his upper and lower teeth, including molars—in other words, after the age of sixteen
months—it is not necessary to mince his food. Providing you
cut it up small, he can eat what the family eats.

And having said that, we come to the problem of your
having, for all practical purposes, to cook twice a day—for
your child at lunchtime and for yourself and your husband in
the evening. (I think for husband-and-wife's sake, you should
avoid eating with your child midday so that Father eats his
meal all by himself in the evening while you just sit and
drink tea.)

Children, you know, do not need complicated recipes. What
is important about their meals is what's in them, not how many
hours have gone into cooking them. Steaming a small portion
of fish in an aluminium colander over his one potato doesn't
take very long. There is no special virtue in cooked green
vegetables for a child; a salad consisting of lettuce, young spinach leaves, or any raw vegetables which the child likes—grated
carrot, chopped celery, tomato, cucumber—will do just as
well.

If you are cooking a casserole for the evening meal, you can
prepare it in the morning so that it is ready by lunchtime.
Then you can give your child a small portion of that and the
rest can be reheated for yourselves—which won't do the
casserole any harm; on the contrary, it will improve the
flavour.

If you aren't doing a casserole and you had fish yesterday,
any of the following will take you twenty minutes' work at

the very outside. Buy 3 to 6 ozs (to allow for shrinkage) of
stewing-steak, pie veal or neck of lamb—these are all cheap cuts
of meat but just as nourishing as best fillet steak—and mince
raw before cooking slowly in gravy in the oven in a covered
fireproof dish. (If you've a fridge, you can safely buy enough
for tomorrow too.)

However, don't run away with the idea that all meat for
young children has to be cooked slowly. Like ours, it depends on
the cut. If you're serving a lamb chop or a piece of veal cutlet or
liver, then fry or grill it as you would your own. But afterwards
mince or chop it, of course. Then make gravy for it by mixing
a minute amount of Marmite (very cheap at your local clinic)
with some vegetable water—yes, I'm coming to the vegetables
—and boiling it up with the meat-juices that have run out
into the pan . . . having first, naturally, drained off the excess
fat. Gravy is a 'must' for toddlers; they nearly all like their
food very moist.

Vegetables: If today's menu is a small potato, one carrot and
three sprouts, let me assure you that you don't have to have
three saucepans on the go. One will do. Toddlers eat their
food mixed up anyway, so that it doesn't matter if the flavour
of sprout gets into the potato or whatever in the cooking. Right
—boil a well-scrubbed potato in its jacket (the goodness sits
mainly just under the skin). When it's half-cooked, add the
sprouts and chopped carrot; this way all the food will be
ready together but the greens won't be mushy and spoilt.

Then put the sprouts and carrot on your child's dish while
you peel the potato and then return it to its saucepan to be
dried and mashed in butter. You'll find that the hot potato,
the boiling gravy and the hot meat are sufficient to warm up
the whole meal to your child's taste.

At weekends there's no problem: he can share your
roast joint or chicken.

Your child's tea should also contain protein: beans, fish,
cheese or egg—for instance, welsh rarebit at teatime on a day
when he ate boiled egg for breakfast. And to ring the changes
for tea: why not baked beans or a little fish occasionally? And
fish doesn't have to be fresh fish; it can even be something
like pilchards or sardines. At teatime and breakfast, use bread-

and-butter, toast or rusk as an addition to his meal, not as the main course.

I am almost always opposed to pudding. Pudding means a lot of unnecessary starch. A piece of cheese and fresh fruit—an apple, for instance, or an orange with the pith and membranes removed—needs no cooking and is much healthier.

You may be thinking that fresh fruit is also a lot dearer than blancmange, fruit jellies and rice pudding. You want to do your best for your child; on the other hand you have to think of your housekeeping money. So to keep costs down, I'd cut out fruit squashes, ice-cream and biscuit snacks between meals.

Teach your child to drink water when he's thirsty; make ice-cream an occasional treat pudding rather than an everyday habit; never introduce him to the idea that the biscuit tin can be raided whenever he feels peckish.

Round about this time your child will probably learn in earnest to feed himself and, in my experience, when he's acquired this skill, he'll become fiercely independent and strongly resent any help. And once he can eat on his own without spreading his food all over himself, his table, and anything else in the neighbourhood, it's a good idea for him to have his meals with the family.

I would recommend a high-chair—it's specially designed for a toddler's comfort and safety, and you can see him (no mean advantage, this) and, more important, he is at the right height to see you. He is at his own table, but at least this is pushed up against the family table; so that once again we are using a mealtime as a social occasion—an occasion in which he participates.

Of course, in different households routines are different. For instance, if your husband comes home after seven o'clock at night, you can't very well keep a one-year-old up so that he can eat with his parents. But he can still have breakfast and/or lunch with *you* and perhaps at weekends he can eat with you both. Yes, I realise that *what* you and your baby eat will be different, but it is still useful if you eat your meals together. We come back to the point that a baby and increasingly a child is a small adult, not somebody from a different planet.

Therefore the more he can share a family activity as important as having meals, the better.

At this stage there is no question of introducing formal table manners. To expect him to handle a knife and fork would be ridiculous; but to expect him to put his food into his mouth as tidily as *he is able* is something else again. This should be taught in a friendly but firm manner, and until he can do this well, you are mistaken in supposing he can eat unaided. And when guests come to table, frankly I feel it is unfair to expect them to watch the off-putting spectacle of a child dribbling poached egg or chocolate cake down his chin. Far better for the learner to eat beforehand on his own—or rather with the one companion, possibly yourself, who is to supervise his feeding. Equally when he eats at a friend's house, I suggest you feed him first.

By the way, if a child who knows perfectly well how to drink properly from a mug, tips his milk upside down, then he doesn't really want it. Take it away from him before he drenches his hair and the floor.

18 months – 5 years

From eighteen months upwards, increasingly it becomes a question of the child eating what and when adults eat. And this brings us to a common difficulty. In a case where you already have a three-year-old and now a new baby, it may be tricky to fit in the main meal for the older child, the two o'clock feed for the baby and a lunch-snack for yourself. Three quite different lots of cooking to do—and your meal and the three-year-old's ideally to be ready at the same time, so that you can sit down together . . .

Well, there is no reason why he can't have soup and scrambled egg, or cheese salad and fruit with you for lunch and his *dinner* meal at 5.30ish. (If you and your husband usually eat sufficiently early, he can actually eat with you.) There's no problem about going straight to bed after food—in fact nature intended us to curl up in our cave immediately after our burnt bearsteak. (If you doubt me, think of your pets: *they* sleep after a meal. Think of Grandpa after Christmas lunch: isn't he having forty winks in the armchair?)

But bear in mind your child shouldn't *bath* within an hour of a big meal. This would be easily solved if you switched his bathtime to morning.

After dentition is complete, food need no longer be cut up finely, just sufficiently for his size of mouth. As his appetite gets larger, always increase the protein in his diet (the meat, eggs and so on) far more than the vegetables and starch. And gradually you will need to stop mixing up his food but serve it instead in separate little mounds—a smaller version, in fact, of your own plate. Children, too, need their food to look appetising. And when he can cope with such a meal all on his own (with an adult doing no more than the cutting up beforehand), *then* is the time for him to transfer from his highchair to a bulky cushion at the dining-table.

Perhaps I ought to say that for most children highly-spiced foods should be avoided; but I have known children who had a positive passion for things like curry, pickled onions and highly-flavoured cheeses. So to some extent be guided by what likes and dislikes your own child has.

Now, all children, however placid they are about eating what's put in front of them, do develop periodic dislikes for certain things. If you accept these fancies calmly, however, the dislike tends to go on to something else—perhaps from greens to mushrooms, and then off mushrooms on to scrambled egg; and then in the end the child likes scrambled egg but dislikes bacon. These phases of disliking a food—for its colour, its texture or its taste—are not serious. Nor is the converse—a passion for a certain food almost to the exclusion of everything else. It might be tomato sauce or corn flakes. Try indulging the passion, but over-indulge it. Tomato sauce three times a day is pretty vile even to the most dedicated sauce taker.

While on the subject of passions, let's talk about the curse of the Seventies—sweets. When I was brought up, sweets were rationed by a strict Mama. For the next generation they were rationed by the Government, but the effect was the same: sweets were not considered an unlimited goody of life. But for today's children they can be, and there are four reasons why this is a very bad thing.

First of all, dental health again. Secondly, your purse.

Sweets are far from cheap. Third: eating sweets between meals ruins the appetite and your child won't manage to finish the meat and vegetables he truly needs. And lastly, it's bad for his character. You and I as adults know that we can't have everything we want any time we want it. I'm not even certain that we'd be happier if we could. Equally, if not more so, this applies to your child. Surely it is wrong for him to pop a toffee in his mouth whenever the fancy takes him, or not to be able to pass a confectioner's without dragging you inside to buy him a quarter of fudge or an ice-lolly?

Of course I'm not saying he must never eat sweets. That's too Victorian. But help him to regard sweets as a family treat —three bars of chocolate for the lot of you to eat during the Sunday walk in the park, or a huge bag of fruit drops for a long car journey—rather than as part of his, and his alone, diet.

You will notice I tend to overdo the sweets when I do hand them round. A dental hygienist assures me that the deposit left by a whole half-pound of sweets eaten on the trot is only minimally worse than that left by a couple. It's the continual, steady eating throughout each day that does the real harm. The advantage of overdoing it works on the same principle as tomato sauce for a week. The child feels ever so slightly fed up with sweets and it may be two or three days before he even wants another. Fine.

I know this because in my own family each of my three children had his own sweet tin. I kept these in a cupboard, and the children asked for their own tin when they wanted a sweet. But they knew very well that once that tin was empty, it stayed empty until the next buying round. It wasn't magically filled every week. And, looking back, it's surprising how often they *didn't* badger me.

Right, they're the sweets you can control. What about those you can't—the ones friends give your child and the ones he buys with his own pocket-money? Well, like we said: sweets are dear. Presumably you're not going to give your under-five-year-old more than 5–10p a week, and that won't buy him a killer dose—not when he's also got to pay for such vital necessities as marbles and save up for yet another little car. Any-

way, for social reasons he may well need to buy sweets sometimes—you know, to win friends and influence other small
people. And this *does* matter to him socially.

As for the sweets he's *given* : this probably depends on how
often it's likely to happen. If Grandma is going to indulge him
every single Sunday, then stop her. But if you spend a once-a-
year afternoon with the wife of your husband's boss and her
spoiled child has a daily bowl of Liquorice Allsorts, you may
decide to ignore the sugar intake today, for the sake of your
husband's career. Oppose her if you dare, of course; but if you
do, you're a better woman than I !

The way to a child's heart is through his stomach . . .
Regretfully that statement is not without exceptions. Your child
has a way of suddenly hating the lunch you've cooked for
him—and not because you've allowed him biscuits or sweets
during the morning, either. Perhaps he's just not hungry today.
I'm against forcing a child to finish food he obviously doesn't
want. But equally I'm very opposed to allowing him to leave
his liver and bacon and eat his ice-cream instead—'I'm not
bread and butter hungry,' type of reasoning.

Very often a child will indicate he doesn't want greens, for
instance, the moment he sees them on his plate. In my own
family we had a golden rule for dealing with this, which you
might at least consider adopting. The rule was very simple.
The instant the child said, 'I don't like that,' we said, 'Splendid—all the more for us,' and it was shared out among the
rest of the family. The child soon found that somehow he was
missing something everybody else enjoyed, and I'd notice that
the next time he'd probably choose to keep his portion.
Although all my children had temporary phases of 'I don't like
fish,' or 'I don't like mince,' or 'I don't like this, that or the
other,' I can honestly say that now they are in their teens and
my elder daughter is a young married woman, they may have
preferences, but all three of them eat whatever is served to
them.

Now, suppose you or your husband do hate something, yet
you reckon your child ought to eat it because it's good for him.
First of all he'll know you dislike it, even if he is only a few
months old at the time. Babies, since they can't understand

verbal communication, are particularly sensitive to attitude and, however much you think you are disguising it, if you are giving him spinach, for example, and you dislike spinach intensely, he'll be aware of it. Don't be surprised if he resists you as firmly as you probably resisted the person who tried to force you to eat spinach. Perhaps it is almost better to avoid giving a child food which you yourself dislike. There are alternatives to spinach—perhaps not with oodles of iron, but with sufficient.

Conversely, you could try our family trick in reverse. Rather delightfully, it worked this way round too. There were many things my husband had never eaten before we met— any form of green vegetable, cooked or uncooked, and yoghurt, flavoured or plain, among others. And I wanted our children to eat both vegetables and yoghurt. Of course, as soon as the children began to eat with us, they realised that Daddy wasn't having some of the good things which we were having. And it could only be explained to them by saying Daddy didn't like those foods because he had never been given them when he was a little boy. But the principle of feeling left out must have worked on him too, because he now enjoys green vegetables and yoghurt as frequently as the rest of us!

Perhaps to end this chapter we ought to talk a little about the subject of table manners. Now, we've discussed feeding problems; if you're having one—however temporary—it is obviously not a logical time to interrupt your child with a 'Not like that, dear'. I mean, it is rather adding insult to injury to make him practise holding his cup elegantly when he's just rejected the milk which is in that cup! The food itself is the vital thing; sophisticated table manners can be successfully instilled in a child after the age-range of this book.

But generally speaking, the earlier manners are taught the more automatic they become. Once your child is approximately two years old, gently but firmly start to correct him. Any habit you are trying to form in your child can be learnt only by constant, patient repetition; so be prepared to say the same thing over and over again. How you want him to put down his knife and fork; whether you want him to eat with a spoon only or whether you want him to eat with a spoon and fork, one held in either hand; stopping him blowing bubbles into his milk—introduce him to the standards you expect in your family, whatever they may be. Table manners vary from household to household just as they vary from country to country. So teach him whatever behaviour you feel comfortable with, not some remote text-book etiquette.

Be warned : if most of the time you allow your child to eat as he pleases—with his hands, by putting food on his head and the wall, using whatever utensils suit his mood—then you cannot suddenly, perhaps because you're visiting friends, expect perfect table manners and scold or even punish him because he doesn't come up to standard. Learning table manners is a slow process. You can't hope for miracles in one day.

Finally I'd like to discuss if it is useful to make a meal the occasion for a story, the sort of story which continues every time the child willingly opens his mouth for the next spoonful and stops when he stops—and all sorts of variations on that theme. The other theory is competition as part of the meal : 'Let's see who can eat this faster, you or I, or you or your brother.' All such activities make a problem out of mealtimes. It is not necessary. It is something which people start in an attempt to distract a child who is temporarily having a difficult phase with his eating—probably just while he's adjusting to new flavours. People think that if they can only get the food into him while he's thinking about something else, they're benefiting him. In my view they are not. On a short-term basis, yes; on a long-term basis they are convincing him that he must have some other interesting activity to compensate for swallowing this unpleasant substance called food. *And eating should be a pleasure*. Regard it as such, and sooner or later your child will too.

CHAPTER TWO

. . . Next to Godliness

THIS CHAPTER is about hygiene—the subject which covers everything from the first time you bath your baby to teaching him how to go to the lavatory by himself.

0 – 15 months

Before you leave hospital or before the midwife leaves your home, you will have been shown how to bath your new baby, and if this is your first baby you will probably feel very clumsy, very inexperienced. All sorts of horrible thoughts like 'What happens if I drop him and he drowns?' will pass through your mind for several days, if not longer, each time you run in the water. First of all, it's highly unlikely he will slither out of your grasp and, even if he does, you just quickly and calmly pick him up again. That's what you're there for.

May I say here that it is unnecessary to buy an expensive baby bath, because your baby will outgrow it very soon. The cheapest plastic bath will do him for the first few months of his life. After that, having a bath in the big bath—and you'll be just the right height to support him in there if you kneel on the bathmat—is much more fun. The big bath offers more space for splashing, and kicking and zooming up and down with Mummy's help. Most babies, after a very few days, look forward to bathtime as one of the pleasure play periods of the day. Incidentally, bathing your baby every day is not essential, particularly if you use an antiseptic foam product like Infacare or Boots' Baby Care. (I favour them because they cut out that chilly business of soaping the baby on your lap beforehand.

34

A quick wash of his face and bottom with cotton wool
and he can get into all that nice warm water. Infacare is also
marvellous for preventing scurf developing, since you wash his
hair with it, too.) You may, of course, *prefer* to give him the
daily splash, but that's a question of pleasure rather than hygiene. The point is : you don't need to feel guilty because you
didn't get around to bathing him today. Twice a day 'topping
and tailing' is adequate for a small baby.

After he can sit up on his own, you will probably introduce all the usual bath toys which family and friends provide.
You and your husband might as well get used to the fact that
for several years to come your bath will be surrounded by ducks,
fishes, boats and weird underwater craft. A plastic shopping
net, hanging on the wall, will keep this aquatic population at
bay.

15 months – 2½ years

The time will come when your baby is no longer a baby but a
small boy or girl who will try to take an active part in washing
himself. I know you can do it much more efficiently and faster
without his help, but your child needs to do things for himself
as early as he's capable.

Admittedly, some children wouldn't dream of touching a
face-flannel or a piece of soap until they're two-and-a-half,
but they are probably only children who don't spend a large
proportion of their lives with other children. It is generally
found that those going to play groups or nursery schools want
to wash themselves earlier than the children who stay at home
with Mother. Also, children who are not the first child in the
family learn to do this sooner, because as a rule they want to
imitate other children rather more than they want to imitate
adults. So perhaps the hardest task is teaching the oldest child
how to be independent. Unconsciously he'll largely teach the
younger ones.

So any time from fifteen months, your child may want to
hold the soap when you wash his hands and face; next he'll
try to wash his own face with the sponge or flannel which, of
course, will drip and soak his shirt or her dress. Nevertheless,
these attempts should not be discouraged, because it is only

when he reaches the point when he wants to do this himself that you can begin to teach him a face flannel can be squeezed so that it isn't dripping wet. Then, when you've got his interest, teach him how to wash his neck and ears. If he's been playing in the sand or out in the garden, introduce him to a soft nail-brush with which to scrub his finger-nails. In any case hand-washing before all meals, and after using the pot, is a must. Keep a spare flannel and a towel in the kitchen, for this reason.

By this time, too, you should have started cleaning his teeth with a child's soft toothbrush. At first you may use just water, but soon he'll need toothpaste. I'd use a flavoured fluoride children's one—it may not have any medicinal advantage over its adult counterpart, but your child will prefer its taste— and *willingness* to have his teeth brushed is half the battle. Show him how to clean his own teeth by demonstrating the correct method, which is not to run the toothbrush backwards and forwards but to run it up and down. Now I come to think about it, our children may be the first generation to do this automatically. We learned too late in life and still have to make a conscious effort to remember the right way: 'Up and down; up and down . . .'

Bear in mind he can't see what you're doing in his mouth, only feel it. His first attempts, therefore, are bound to be clumsy and slow. You may find at first that you will have to clean his teeth properly and then give him the toothbrush to do them again. Always do it this way round—never let him fiddle with his teeth first and then correct him. That's crushing. It is like a school-teacher having her young pupils write in their exercise books and then she goes round and, as it were, invali-dates their work by showing them the proper way. Far better for her to put something on the blackboard to be copied as well as her pupils are able.

$2\frac{1}{2}$ – 5 years

On the subject of general hygiene, I would like to mention the child with a runny nose. There is nothing more revolting, nothing that makes your child less acceptable socially to his own friends, to adults, even to his father, than a constant sniff and a trail of catarrh. Always remember that Father's identification with the child is not as intense as yours, which is why you take for granted cleaning him when he has been sick, washing his bottom when he has had his bowels open; while Father —much as he loves his child—is liable to be repulsed. And of all things there is nothing so repulsive as a child whose nose is perpetually running for weeks on end.

Until your child is approximately two-and-a-half to three years old, wiping his nose is something you have to do. Now, there is nothing more unhygienic than a small or large cotton handkerchief. Handkerchiefs are not only germ-carriers; they are lethal. If you wish to prolong a cold—anyone's cold—use handkerchiefs. But if you want to get rid of a cold, use tissues which are immediately disposed of by being burnt or flushed down the toilet. If tissues—especially during a period when the whole family has colds—are too expensive, perhaps instead you have some old sheeting which you could cut up into pieces approximately the size of a handkerchief. Use them and dispose of them. Don't wash them and use them again.

From about the age of two-and-a-half a child should be taught the muscular skill of blowing his nose. Curious though it may seem, this isn't something he finds out naturally. (The proof of this is that in communities where no one bothers to teach children to be socially acceptable, children of seven, eight or nine are still running around with runny noses.) And the act of blowing is very difficult to describe, so the following game may well be a help to you.

You take an ordinary washing-up bowl of water, and you float on it a feather—a small feather: perhaps a bird's feather you have found or a feather from a pillow. You then put your hand firmly over your mouth and you attempt to move the feather by blowing air at it through your nose, and this action is exactly the same action which is used when you blow your nose. Obviously, you invite the child to come and watch. (Don't do this as a punishment for having a runny nose, but as a game. And naturally choose a time when your child—or you —hasn't got a cold.) He'll think it fun and want to join in. Perhaps you will need to put your hand over his mouth to begin with, until he gets the idea that the only way you can do this is by having the mouth firmly closed and not allowing

air to pass out through the mouth. And as soon as your child
has learnt how to move the feather, he has learnt how to blow
his nose.

Sooner or later your child will ask you why we go through
this rigmarole called washing. You could say because it com-
bats illness, but that sounds awfully dull. There's nothing so
boring as health to a healthy person; it's only sick people who
are obsessed with it. And I am assuming your child is well.
I'd take the attitude that we wash because it's nice to be clean.

It is infinitely preferable to associate cleanliness with pleasant sensation, 'it's nice to be clean', rather than if you associate
dirt with unpleasant ones—having to wash because dirt is
nasty. Besides, dirt is not necessarily nasty; it depends on what
you're doing. Sand's dirty; but if your child is playing in sand,
then this dirty substance is nice. It is only when he tries to mix
the sand with food that it becomes undesirable. If you are gardening and your hands are working in soil, it is not nasty; on
the contrary, it is very pleasant. It again becomes something to
be avoided if you come in and begin to cook without washing your hands thoroughly first. So press home the association
of cleanliness with niceness and get away from the idea of 'It's
nasty to be dirty'.

0 – 1 years
Very much the same thing applies when you are changing
nappies. I hear many young mothers when they're talking to
their babies about their soiled nappies say how nasty it is having to clean him, rather than the much more positive approach
of 'How nice it is to be clean'. The less nastiness in verbal comment and attitude over excretion, the better. After all, it is just
a normal bodily function.

Incidentally, many adults imagine that children are born
with an instinctive revulsion to their own excreta; this is
not so. On the contrary, many psychiatrists believe that for
babies *producing* excreta—in other words, the contents of
soiled nappies—is making a gift for Mother; and if Mother's
response to that gift is revulsion in her attitude or what she
says, the child will be aware of it and, at best, merely puzzled,
at worst, very hurt. So do please try to control your acquired

attitude of how nasty this is, and you will be benefiting your child's emotional health—quite apart from feeling less revolted yourself.

Now, on the question of nappies . . . As you know, there are many different types of nappies on the market. There are the ordinary conventional square terry towelling nappies; there are now shaped nappies—a little more expensive, these, but useful because they fit more snugly and you avoid getting lumpy bits on the baby's hips and between his legs—and there are disposables. On disposable nappies, I can only say 'Just watch your plumbing', because plumbing, certainly in Britain, was not designed to take the vast quantity of disposable material with which we tend to overload it.

Disposable nappies certainly have their value, particularly when travelling—even if it is only travelling for the day—but as a permanent solution to the problem of nappy washing, I wouldn't really recommend them, because they are not as comfortable as towelling. Moreover, they are not as absorbent. Mothers who use disposable nappies all the time have to change their babies twice as often.

'Ah,' you argue, 'but you're not the one who has to wash the towelling ones.' True; but the myths about the toils of nappy washing should be a thing of the past. No one should have to boil nappies. No one nowadays should have to have lines and lines of dripping nappies hanging over their heads in the kitchen and bathroom. Not in the 1970s. In any chemist's you will find a substance like the proprietary Napisan, which was specially designed to sterilise and remove the stains from babies' nappies. (It is also ideal for your baby's whites—sheets, bibs, cotton suits or dresses.) The instructions on how to use it are clearly given on every container. Incidentally, these containers—providing they've been thoroughly washed—make excellent storage jars afterwards thanks to their very good snap-on-lids. The only thing you need in addition is a large plastic bucket with a well-fitting lid, and in hard-water areas a chemical water-softener.

Now, nappies which have been soaking in Napisan usually don't need further washing; but if you do find that some which were heavily soiled still have some stains, then wash them in something like Persil or pure soap flakes. (A word of warning : detergents and biological washing powders may produce nappy rash. Don't ever use them for baby clothes and nappies however well they work on things like tea-towels, pillow-cases and husband's shirts.)

All nappies need is thorough rinsing and by thorough I mean they need rinsing-wringing, rinsing-wringing, rinsing-wringing—whether you wring by hand, whether you have a wringer, or whether you have the modern and far more convenient method : a spin-drier. Electrical shops and indeed the electricity companies often have reconditioned small spin-driers fairly cheap and, now it's not so easy to get down to the launderette, you might think it worth your while investing in one. Or you could look on the noticeboard at your infant welfare clinic. There are often second-hand ones offered for sale among the prams and baby-walkers.

If you do have a garden, it's a good idea to put out all your baby's washing for a little while and have the fresh air blowing through it. This makes nappies softer, sweeter-smelling, and fresh air does combat germs. For mothers without gardens, I would recommend that occasionally, especially on wet days, you use the tumble drier at the local launderette.

The old-fashioned idea that nappies have to be ironed we no longer need to discuss. I don't think there is any mother in the 1970s who will insist on ironing her nappies every day. And, of course, with all the new drip-dry materials, the task of coping with a baby's laundry is also considerably reduced.

By the way, you can avoid the worst soiling on nappies by using one of the disposable nappy liners (available at any chemist's or baby shop) inside the towelling nappy. Then when you next change your baby, you simply throw the soiled liner down the toilet, and the towelling nappy will still be clean. Of course, the majority of the time the liner, too, won't be soiled, merely wet. In this case save yourself some money and stick it in the Napisan pail with the other nappies. Although nappy liners look like fragile paper tissues, they are in fact far stronger. They withstand washing and even spin drying quite merrily, and can be used two or three times before they finally disintegrate.

Before we leave the subject of nappies, I'd like to discuss 'marathons', the one-way traffic nappies—in other words, wet passes through them and cannot get back again and so the surface next to the baby's skin remains dry. They are a nappy liner in as much as they go inside the terry-towelling nappy, but their life is as long as the towelling one's. They're ideal for nights when you don't have regular opportunities for changing your baby, for they keep his bottom and the whole area round his groins and genitals free from rash and irritation.

Incidentally, do sponge him with clean warm water *every* time he's changed, even when the nappy has not been soiled; because although the skin looks clean, the salts from urine which still cling to the skin surface can cause irritation as much as excreta can. Dry him thoroughly. You don't have to use towels; you can use tissues or cheap cotton wool for this purpose. Pat on baby powder, or perhaps a little baby cream (I can recommend Morsep) if you can see the beginnings of any soreness—watch out for this particularly when your baby is teething as dentition often causes upsets. Prevention is better than cure here. Nappy rash can be very uncomfortable and makes the baby fretful and you too by the end of the day. More than likely you're both suffering needlessly. But there are babies who have specially sensitive skins, and in the case of persistent irritation you really should show it to your health visitor or doctor.

1 – 2 years

This brings us to the question of for how long do you go on using nappies? That depends on your child. It doesn't really depend on you, but you can help him to give up the need for nappies when he is ready. Fortunately, the influence of psychiatric research has brought it to common knowledge that early toilet-training is undesirable. It places a strain on the nervous system, because it makes the baby anxious about something which he can't really control.

Although there's no suggestion anywhere that mothers who used early toilet-training punished their children if they didn't succeed, the fact that they were pleased when their three- or four-month-old did use the pot instead of soiling his nappy brought its own stresses.

As a mother you have probably noticed already that your baby attempts to please you, and if he fails in this he will be worried. So please don't ask him to do something which is beyond him because he's simply too young to have control of his excretory muscles.

I'm not preaching from above. I am one of those mothers myself who attempted early toilet-training on my first child. My elder daughter, who is now a mother herself, used to say to people when she was in her teens that she was her mother's experiment, and she was right because one of my experiments on her—because I firmly believed that this was the thing to do —was early toilet-training. I succeeded, too, apparently. I could proudly announce that by the time my daughter was fourteen months old, I no longer needed nappies for her except at night. She still now has tensions about going to the lavatory.

With my second and third children I was less martial and they, in turn, were far less fraught.

Somewhere between a year and eighteen months—decide when your own child is ready—introduce the pot. This works better if it is done as a game at first, rather than as something very serious and very important and very needful of success. So originally use the pot unrelated to its real purpose—I remember we used ours as a container for bricks; we carried it from here to there; we played games with it where we bowled it from one end of the room to the other; we wore it as a hat. And only gradually did the pot go to its rightful place beside the lavatory, where it then stayed. Children are conservative by nature and like to learn where things live. They don't like having things which they're accustomed to seeing in one place suddenly in another. So we as it were learnt that the pot's place of residence was in the bathroom.

Then finally came the day when I took the child to the bathroom, removed his nappy and sat him on the pot. Of course, the child was puzzled and had no idea what to do. And then I found that if I made this sitting on the pot coincide with my own visit to the lavatory, the child discovered slowly by imitation what was supposed to happen in this pot. If the very idea of this embarrasses you, for your child's sake, do overcome it. Reason it out logically and you'll find there's no reason for embarrassment.

Naturally I praised the child when he first succeeded and for a number of occasions afterwards, but I feel strongly that excessive praise is bad. A normal 'Well done', 'good boy' or 'good girl', 'that's it' is enough. In the course of repeating this over and over again, making no comment whatsoever when I took off his wet nappy and therefore he didn't succeed in the pot because he'd already done it—or more—in his nappy, he quickly and very willingly began to co-operate.

My children also learnt what the pot was called. Actually it is not unusual for children who are trained in this way to include the word 'pot', which is easy to say, among their earliest words. They say 'pot' when they want to go to the lavatory, and you down tools and dash. Though some children learn this much earlier, you can expect your child to ask for the pot before he excretes into his nappy by about the age of two. In fact the more calmly you can treat toilet-training, the easier the process will be. And if you avoid anxiety or excessive praise, it will never occur to your child to use his pot as a weapon— performing obediently when you're in favour, using his nappy when he's cross with you.

Pot points to ponder.

We should consider what exactly we are trying to teach a child when we speak of toilet-training. In the first place we are helping him to experience something quite new to him.

1. That his motions or urine are removed as soon as he has passed them.
2. That this is apparently linked with Mother's approval.
3. Approval is nice; therefore the child will deliberately try to create the happening which brings the approval.
4. *Incidentally* he will find out how to control his bladder and bowel excretion.

When you first show your child the 'how and what' of a pot, it is easier to get some results into the pot if you coincide your

attempt with the time when you know he usually has a bowel
motion, such as about half an hour after breakfast. Also it's
worth having a try each time you have his nappy off to change
him—especially when he's just woken up in the morning or
after his rest.

Now, I appreciate that you can go through this drill for
weeks on end with a 19-month-old, regularly sitting him on
his pot while you yourself go to the lavatory, and he'll never
once get the message. Yet you think you could catch him if
the pot was in the room where he was playing. Fair enough.
Then *temporarily* and strictly while you're alone together, take
the pot to him—or in summer even out into the garden while
your child plays without a nappy.

And once he is 'clean' (I hate that term) and at least twice
a day will also pass water into his pot, stop using nappies in the
daytime and put him in trainer pants instead. With these, the
whole toilet-training rigmarole is easier.

Potty-chairs are not potty training; nor is leaving a child on
the pot for half an hour or longer. There is then no connection
between the purpose of sitting on the pot and the result, which
considering the time factor is virtually inevitable. In this case
the child is not performing the act of excretion deliberately but
is merely undergoing the endurance test of sitting there long
enough. (I've heard some mothers complain their children have
emptied their pots on the floor or around the walls. I suspect
such children were victims of an-hour-on-the-pot, and this was
their protest or bored reaction. Under the circumstances, who
can blame them ! So five minutes at the very most.)

For some children even brief visits to the lavatory are a bore.
A small toy which can be manipulated while sitting on the pot
may make him more willing, even eager, to go there. You could
keep such a toy alongside his pot. Do not bring a full size dolls
house or a complete train set up from the living-room with him.

If your child resists your effort to seat him on the pot—he
cries, stiffens, clings to you—IT'S TOO SOON. Your child isn't
stupid; if you put his bare bottom on this hard plastic thing,
he'll understand vaguely what you want of him and realise
that it's something he knows he can't provide. That distresses
him. So put the pot away for a month and then try again.

2 – 3 years

I know some little girls who simultaneously learnt how to manage to be without nappies at night as well as in the day, but they are not many; and boys very often need nappies at night for much, much longer. It is not unusual for four to five-year-old boys to need nappies at night for complete safety.

For night-training all you do is put the child on the pot at his bedtime and again at your own bedtime. You may or may not have succeeded in having a dry nappy in between, but sit him on the pot regardless to establish a habit. There is no point in potting a child every two hours during the night. I have known some mothers do this, and they achieve nothing— just a tired child and a tired mother. Part of the trick of learning control is to be able to maintain it during a longer and longer period of time; and whilst in the daytime it's not unusual for a child to need to go on the pot every two hours, to encourage him to do this at *night* is really working against toilet-training.

There may be a short period when your child succeeds in going through the night but wakes at six o'clock positively 'bursting', and until he can pull his pyjama trousers down or lift a nighty—if you're using nighties for a little girl—and sit himself on the pot, I'm afraid you will have to get up and help him. But take heart; it doesn't last long.

Now, on night-training there are a few factors to be considered. One of them is that some children will continue to need a nappy while they are being given a nappy. There comes a point for every mother when she wants to put her child in pyjamas without a nappy—and she should let him know he hasn't any nappy—and risk that these pyjamas will be wet in the morning. It hardly needs to be said that the mattress should be adequately protected in a waterproof cover, so that if the child does not remain dry, there isn't much harm done —only a pair of pyjamas and a sheet to wash. And the following night maybe you'll be luckier.

Your child may need an incentive to help him stay dry. Perhaps some new pyjamas which he himself thinks are attractive is sufficient. Or maybe a change of environment—he's gone to stay with a favourite relative—may do the trick.

But the important thing is that if your child is normally

happy during the daytime, he plays and doesn't show any anxiety symptoms—like sitting for hours sucking his fingers compulsively—the fact that he is still wet at three, four or even five years old should not cause you to fear he will remain a bed-wetter for the rest of his life. If you're particularly concerned, by all means mention it to the clinic or your doctor; but ten to one, either will only repeat what I've said. Moreover, even if you do have a persistent bed-wetter, he will probably suddenly be cured, often by the most amazing means.

My son, when he was nine years old, had a friend who was still a persistent bed-wetter. Well, we went on holiday to Belgium, and while in Brussels we visited the famous statue of Mannikinpis—the little boy who is making water into a fountain. My son was very fascinated with this statue and in one of the nearby souvenir shops he asked to buy one of the little replicas. 'I want to give it to my friend,' he told me. 'It'll help him.' Heaven knows how Nicholas knew it, but his friend has not wetted his bed from the day he received his Mannikinpis!

We all know that there are many words—none of which are particularly nice—which describe the action of passing water or having a bowel motion. I personally don't think that any of them is required. There is no reason for a child to tell you what he has done or what he is about to do. To say that he is doing jobs No 1 or No 2, and all the other words for this, is really not necessary; and your child will use such words only if you do. Why not teach him simply to say: 'Potty, Mummy' or 'I want to go to potty', or even just 'pot'. This is not a matter of embarrassment or prudery on my part, but rather that our language doesn't have suitable words for a child to use. Besides, we as adults don't hold long conversations about the act; if we say anything, we merely say we're popping upstairs to the lavatory; we don't go into lengthy descriptions about what we're going to do when we get there!

Now, I admit that, in spite of the fact that *you* haven't taught your child any such words, when he goes to nursery school or play group later on, he may well pick one up. Hard luck. Take consolation in the fact it won't be very deep-seated and he won't use the word very frequently if you don't use it at home.

I would strongly advise that a pot is not carried about all

over the house. Once the pot has found its home next to the lavatory, it ought to stay there. It doesn't need to be brought into the sitting-room because your child can't cope with his pants; your child should call you and you should go to the lavatory with him. He also doesn't have to bring the pot out to show you he has finished. He need only call you so that you can empty the pot and rearrange his clothes for him to go off to play again.

3 – 5 years

The transition from pot to lavatory is one that happens gradually and to some extent is related to your child's height. For a little boy to learn how to pass water standing up, for instance —and particularly how to do it into the lavatory rather than into the pot—requires that he be tall enough to reach over the lavatory comfortably, or is able to cope with a footstool. By the way, you'll probably have to rope in your husband here; this is obviously a lesson that has to be taught by a man.

For little girls, you can buy a child's toilet seat which lodges over the lavatory and teach her to sit on this rather than a pot. Certainly you then no longer have the bother of emptying a pot, and it makes the transition to the proper lavatory far simpler. But do avoid letting the child's toilet seat 'live' on the lavatory permanently; it can throw a guest to be confronted by this contraption unexpectedly!

Perhaps in conclusion I should say that although we are apparently so permissive about toilet-training, in that we don't expect our baby under a year even to attempt it, this doesn't mean it's unimportant. There is a definite value in teaching your child to use first the pot and then the lavatory, instead of the nappy—or, worse, instead of running about without a nappy and passing water and bowel motions anywhere he pleases. I have actually seen this in certain trendy homes and I've been assured by the 'progressive' parents it was one way of allowing the child complete freedom and avoiding repression. To my mind it is also a way of not fulfilling one's duty as a parent, because it is up to parents to teach their child to fit into society, and society expects its members to use the lavatory. So we have a responsibility here—a responsibility which we carry out with love.

CHAPTER THREE

A Member of the Family

IF YOU'RE reading this book during pregnancy or perhaps even in hospital before you go home, it may not have occurred to you that what was a relationship for two people, has become a family. Not only are you now a mother as well as a wife, but you are also a member of a new family unit—and so is your son or daughter, who is possibly at this moment in his cot in the nursery. You should acknowledge this family factor now, otherwise your child will remain an outsider, an intruder in a twosome household—and that's sad for him, and even sadder for you. We must also be very clear about the fact that the family does consist of at least three of you. Your husband's role is just as important as yours. It's important from your husband's point of view just as much as from your child's and your own. A father who feels that his job has been accomplished because you now have what you wanted—which was a baby— is liable to feel excluded from the intense and intimate relationship which will develop between you and your child. No father is ever as emotionally and biologically involved with his children as a mother; he cannot be. But his need and desire to do what is useful, healthy and what makes the child happy— that's something else again. It gives your child the sense of security only two parents can provide, and it is of deep emotional value to your husband as well.

Of course, the degree to which fathers are willing to assist in the practical upbringing of a child, particularly in the first three months, is variable. Some men take to feeding the baby, bathing him, changing nappies, generally acting as your other

half when you are busy, just like ducks to water. Many men
are very proud to take out their heir in the pram on Sunday
mornings or on a summer week-night when you're busy getting
the dinner; but it is not an indication that a father loves his
child less because—due to his upbringing and the attitudes he
has as a result of it—he just can't bring himself to help in this
practical way to any signficant extent. The more you bully him,
the more you insist on having your husband do the things
which you know other people's husbands do, the more resentful and resistant he will be. You can only persuade him gently;
you can only ask and request—and appreciate, however little
or however much he does do.

Perhaps he would prefer doing something about the dinner
while you deal with the baby. Thought about that? Perhaps
he genuinely feels a little ham-fisted, fearing he might hurt the
baby because he isn't really sure what he's handling. Men often
feel hesitant about plunging in and playing things by ear;
whilst a woman will say: 'Well, all right, I'll have a go at this.
I don't know that I'm much good at it, but I'll try.' In areas
which have for centuries been the field of women, men tend to
be wary—not all men, but many men.

You may also remember that the father of a first baby
especially may resent the amount of time which you now have
to spend with the baby which you once spent with him. He's
discovering you far more in your role as a mother and much
less in your role as the wife he married. His misses your constant
companionship and he feels a bit put out about it. This is
understandable and something quite different from the almost
sexual jealousy which some men feel over their child and wife.
Here I would just like to say that if you notice your husband is
at all disturbed when you are breast-feeding, make it your business to take the baby into another room—into the bedroom
perhaps or into the baby's room. I know it's a violation of that
idealised picture of togetherness you had of the three of you;
but it's just too bad. If your husband doesn't like seeing you
breast-feed, it's highly unlikely you can talk him round. Don't
fight about it; just quietly remove the source of the agitation.

A baby's attitude to his father depends largely on how well
he knows him. Babies don't automatically love their fathers;

they don't automatically love their mothers. They will love those with whom they have contact, and this means physical contact too. You may be planning all sorts of glorious things for his future, but your baby cannot know that he's loved unless he's cuddled, spoken to, played with, and has his needs attended to. And if he doesn't feel loved, he cannot learn to love in return.

So if Father is to be loved, is to have anything but merely the role of the man who provides the money, he should spend time with his baby—and I mean by that from the earliest days onwards: preferably from the birth itself. He should talk to the baby, play with him, hold him.

Perhaps a good hint on how to encourage your husband to form this active relationship with his new baby, is not to stand over him giving directions on how to do whatever it is he is doing. Even though he may be doing it badly, even though he's not doing it the way you've been taught to do it in hospital, go into another room and leave these two members of the family—your family—to carry on with getting to know each other. Your baby will suffer a far greater wound from having a distant stranger for a father than he ever will from having a nappy pin prick his thigh!

And the other 'don't', the important 'don't', is not to use Father as the Big Bad Wolf—never. Because your small baby is crying a lot or being irritable one day, to say—even in fun— 'You wait till Daddy comes home; he'll deal with you' is creating a nasty concept which later on he may unconsciously accept. So beware.

It is interesting and very touching to watch the different relationship which develops between a father and son—even when the son is under three months old—and a father and daughter. With his son, he is a pal. They romp; they chat; they play football in the garden. But with his daughter he is tender and protective. At the risk of being considered way-out, I should like to state that it is generally acknowledged there is an element of an unconscious sexual attraction between father and daughter, just as there is between mother and son. Nothing to get worked up about; it isn't abnormal or wrong. I mention it only because, once you are aware of it, it explains so much. It explains why your own father described your perfectly presentable boy friend as 'a long-haired nit', and why mother-in-law problems exist. Yes : it is not for nothing that little girls can often get whatever their heart desires out of Father, and that mothers have been known for centuries to be the people who've ruined their sons with their spoiling.

The next people who are in the family unit are older brothers and sisters. We are now speaking, of course, of a family where the new baby is not the first child.

Since women have been able to plan their families fairly accurately, a tradition has grown up of the 'two-year gap'. In other words : one aims to conceive the second baby when the first child is fifteen months. This may be revolutionary thinking, but I seriously question the value of having two children with an age-difference of only two years.

During my 'Preparation for Motherhood'—psychoprophylaxis—classes, I was always stressing the importance of not lifting heavy things off the floor . . . especially without first bending the knees and stooping down slowly. And my mothers protested that they *lived* with heavy objects who continually, and often suddenly, required to be lifted off the floor—in other words, their eighteen-month-old toddlers ! And apart from the danger to her poor old back, a pregnant woman shouldn't ideally be coping with the relentless physical work involved in bringing up a child of under two-and-a-half. Once a child is over that age, he may well be exhausting but at least he'll play for an hour while his mother rests on the sofa; he doesn't have to have nappies and clothes washed on a day when she's feeling giddy and sick. You see my point ?

On the coming pages I'm going to discuss 'jealousy problems' over a new baby. Bear in mind a two-year-old is still something of a baby himself. In all probability he'll still wear nappies at night; he'll still require a lot of help with feeding; he'll still need to be dressed. So he may well feel he's too little to be 'replaced' and regard with hostile suspicion the picture of Mummy holding someone else. A three-year-old actively wants to be independent; moreover, he appreciates to some degree the advantages of having a sister or brother. He may even nag you to have a baby like the one Auntie Peggy's got . . .

Yes, you argue, but children of three or four years apart are not companions for each other. Admittedly, this is true. But let's be logical about how long that companionship lasts when the gap is closer. If the children are of opposite sexes, I give it four years at the very most. And even at that, I know many brothers and many sisters who are more adversaries than friends! All is far happier if they don't see too much of each other during the hours of daylight, and instead have their own separate playmates.

And what about the advantage of 'getting the baby period of your life over quickly'? Well, suppose you have three children, at spaces of two years: then from the beginning of your first pregnancy till your last child's third birthday takes nearly eight years—eight years of milk, nappies, pots and squalls. Suppose you married in your early twenties and started your family soon afterwards, then those eight years are your youth. I quite realise that if you have those same three children at spaces of three-and-a-half years, it takes eleven years—even longer but at least between each child you and your husband have had a year's break from pregnancy and babies.

Personally I found this vastly preferable. You may not. I'm just asking you not to rush into this two-year thing without due consideration of these factors.

Talking of the size of your family, I would say that it is certainly beneficial to have more than one child. The only child is often a lonely one. He doesn't learn about the rough and tumble of everyday living so naturally because he is surrounded by considerate adults; thus it comes as a bit of a shock to him as a schoolboy to discover he has to defend himself against unwarranted attack. And of course—owing to the fact you have much more time—it is far easier, far more tempting, to over-indulge an only child. So if it is medically and accommodation-wise possible, it might be better to have a larger family.

How much larger is for you and your husband to decide. But I would warn you that to be a good mother to more then four children requires positive dedication and a very special sort of marriage; moreover providing clothes, meals, fares and a hundred-and-one other essential things for six or so children costs an awful lot of money.

People have attempted to prepare older children for the arrival of the new baby in various ways. I think most of them failed because they didn't appreciate the role of a child in the family well enough. For example, there's a favourite dodge of telling the child that a new baby is coming for *him*. In fact I have been informed by little boys and girls of three and four that *they* were having a baby sister or brother. All works splendidly until the baby is actually born. Then there's trouble. The older child very soon realises that this new property of his isn't something with which he can do whatever he assumed he was going to do with a new toy. Mother and Father won't allow it. He will also find that his new toy is passive, and it needs things which the owner, for whom the baby was brought, cannot provide. It needs to be fed, for instance, and the owner can't do this—at least, not without considerable adult assistance. It doesn't seem to want to play the games brother or sister may want to play. And it doesn't make the sort of responses a a three- or four-year-old or even a two-year-old expects from a playmate.

Thus I feel it is much, much better to explain to an older child that the new baby is coming to *join the family*; he or she is going to live with us and be a part of the family. After all, one would expect far less from a member of the family than one would from a present one thought was exclusively one's own.

So the child won't be *disappointed* in the baby, you think, but he'll still be jealous . . . Think about this coolly and logically. He will only be jealous if he fears you don't love him as much. And if he's good reason to think that, then you—not he—are the one who needs the psychiatrist!

Parents who watch for 'jealousy symptoms' tend to get them. Whereas a girl I met recently had never heard about 'difficulties with an older child' and therefore didn't expect any when her baby arrived. . . . Not a moment's trouble in that direction has she experienced.

I can honestly say that my own three children never expressed overt hostility or jealousy towards the new baby in each case. The only thing I ever did to sweeten the pill of 'Well, there is another person here now, and we'll all have to join in to help look after him because he's small' is that I had the baby bring a 'hello gift' for his older brother and sisters. The gift doesn't have to be anything expensive, but it must be bought and correctly labelled in advance, and be presented to the older child when he is introduced to the new member of the family.

There is a brigade of parents who have always done this, only the gift is specifically a doll—'your new baby, dear, like Mummy's new baby'. I don't really go along with that because, as you know, I am opposed to '*Mummy's new baby*' in the first place. He's the family's new baby and not a piece of property at that. If your toddler's dream thing is a Teddy or a doll for its own sake, then fine—give him one. But the present may equally be something quite mad like a game of Ludo or a cricket bat or a football. Make it whatever your child wants.

In the case of my own second daughter, Merle, who happened to like babies, when her baby brother came we did give her a glove puppet in the form of a baby. She did everything she could with this puppet. She couldn't bath it because that would have been very traumatic for the puppet, since it was soft and wouldn't have taken very kindly to being thrown in the water. But she did breast-feed it and was very annoyed because the baby never seemed to be taking enough, she told me! She also kicked it, threw it, and it lost its hands several times in the first week it arrived. It became a sort of combination of 'My new baby . . . my new doll' and also a football to kick around. Whether or not she worked out what certain psychologists might call unconscious regressions on it, I don't know and I'm not really very bothered. The important thing is : she didn't show any apparent hostility towards the new baby.

Now, it's just possible that you'll do everything I recommend and your older child—because of his nature, or because of his unusual dependence on you—will still be seriously jealous. He may try to hurt the baby—stop this (preferably with a tact-ful 'Stroke him gently' rather than 'Mind his eyes!') for his own sake as much as the baby's. If he succeeds in bashing little sister with his train, he'll only hate himself in addition to the rest of the world, and the bash won't have removed the baby from his home. Alternatively, he may try to be a baby again himself—wanting a bottle or refusing to talk. Indulge him if you *have* to, but be sure he knows you love him just as much as you ever did, and it will soon pass off. But, as I say, twenty to one he'll accept the new member of the family as philosophically, perhaps even as proudly as you and your husband do.

So a child won't inevitably be jealous simply because biologically and emotionally he has to share you with another small person. But what about your *time*—those hours which were once exclusively his? Well, when a woman is having her second baby, she is much more expert at the practical things like changing nappies, doing up the pram reins, deciding what her child should wear on a warm, rainy day . . . Thus she will spend less time on the purely physical taking care of the new baby than she did on her first.

So you will have that much more time to use. And very often you can tend to both your children at the same time—guessing the older one's favourite colour while you purée the new baby's dinner. On certain occasions the baby may not be able to be picked up when he wants to be, because you're playing bowls with Stephen. On the other hand Stephen will just have to accept you can't play Snap just now because you're bathing the baby.

Of course, Stephen may like to join in with the bathing. But don't count on it. The extent to which I'd advise you to encourage an older child to help with the new baby depends very much on the personality of the child. Some little girls especially love to help; other children are just not interested.

Also, there are times when it is not desirable to have the older one there. For instance, while *feeding* the new baby you ought to have your attention on him and not divided by being Mummy and teacher to your toddler—not at the same moment. So there is something to be said for having the older child occupied with his zoo or something while you are attending to the baby.

But usually this joining in works as an occasional thing when the older child clearly says 'I want to help . . .' but it doesn't work as a general policy. Other things apart, the new baby will soon become an awful bore to this child who is expected to have sombre daily duties and responsibilities—like holding the soap-dish and fetching clean nappies!

By and large don't worry too much about this question of

divided loyalties. I think you will find your day falls quite naturally into times when you're with the baby, times when you're
with the older one and times when you can be with both your
children together. And I hope there will still be periods—probably the evenings—for you to be a wife. Not to mention the
odd little chunk to be just yourself—to play badminton, to
visit a girl friend or to stand on your head if that pleases you.
Yes. I mean it. All mothers have to learn that they can be many
things to many people almost at the same time, and that they
can divide the time they thought they didn't have even further!

From the baby's point of view, there are a number of advantages to not being the first which outweigh the disadvantages.
As we mentioned in our chapter on hygiene, second and third
and fourth children learn physical skills like holding a cup and
using the lavatory at an earlier age than a first baby, because
they make a tremendous effort to be grown-up, like the older
child. Later on, they won't resist going to nursery school or
proper school because this seems a sort of goal: '*I* now go to
school, too.'

And the games of older brothers and sisters are tremendously
fascinating for a baby or toddler to watch. Mind you, see that
he doesn't interfere with the pleasures of the older child. Don't
assume that because he is sixteen months and his older brother
and sister are three, they can play together. The frequent observation—'They're both small children; let's put them together
to play'—is a wrong one, because the three-year-old very often
has games which the younger child doesn't understand. He
has made a house with his bricks, and the toddler knocks it
down simply because he doesn't know what else to do. So there
is a lot to be said for keeping them in separate game areas—in
other words, occupying them independently of each other.

When the children are between three and five years, they
will probably play together reasonably happily. Of course
they'll fight. All young creatures fight in the course of play, and
punishment in such a case really must be kept to an absolute
minimum. I always said 'Until they draw blood I'll keep away',
and it's probably a good rule; because although somebody
might punch somebody and somebody else might push somebody back, as long as neither child feels that he can gain paren-

tal attention by being the victim, very little actual damage is done. It's necessary for a child to learn sooner or later that things can be mighty unfair and that this is something he has to sort out for himself. But although I don't like the tell-tale-tit, you may have a child who needs to be listened to so that he can pour out his grievances; but that doesn't mean you have to go into action upon them.

Of course, sometimes you *have* to intervene and be judge. For instance, a particular toy is wanted by two children at the same time, and you feel it isn't right that the bigger one—because of his superior strength—should always win; nor that the smaller one—because he's the baby—should always be indulged. Try taking the toy away altogether. The bone of contention is then removed, and they both hate you; but at least they no longer hate each other. A great bond : a common enemy.

I think while we're talking about the baby as a new member of the family, we might consider whereabouts he should live. And since he spends a lot of his first six months asleep, let's begin with where to put the cot. May I make an earnest plea that, whenever it is possible, no new baby should sleep in the same room as his parents?

There are several reasons for this, one of them is the fact that mothers are liable to be anxious and to want 'to just have a look at him' all the time—or, worse, to lean over and pick him up. This can be lethal because Mother is tired when she cuddles the baby and she is likely to lie down on her bed . . . and fall asleep. Babies have been suffocated that way. But even if your baby's cot is at the other end of the bedroom, nevertheless you will be very conscious of the breathing you can hear, and young babies do snuffle and grunt and make all sorts of noises in their sleep. Thus it will disturb you, and ultimately it will disturb the baby. Anxiety is transmitted to the baby even though it is not verbalised.

You must always remember that a baby almost knows what we are thinking regardless of what we do with our faces and our voices. He has to know. He cannot biologically be exposed to living in a situation where he is totally unable to receive communication; therefore he is ultra-sensitive to the emotions of others. For precisely this reason he would be aware of the sexual relationship between his parents, and this is to his disadvantage. It is also, of course, not conducive to a free flow of intimacy between husband and wife to have the baby there.

So if you do have any other room, put the baby in it. Believe me: he's tougher than he looks. He is not going to die before the dawn just because he's alone in there! Equally, he should be within 'hearing' reach—just in case. So if you yourselves sleep in the West Wing of your stately home, don't put your baby in the East Wing! Incidentally, it's perfectly all right for him to sleep in a room with his older brothers and sisters. Most toddlers sleep very deeply and a baby who wakes up during the night—providing he's not allowed to lie there and cry for two hours—will generally not disturb them.

And babies should not be allowed to lie and cry for two hours. The theory that a new baby will expect to be lifted during the night if you lift him once, is an old-fashioned one. Any tiny baby who needs food or drink or just comfort during the night should have it. If this is correctly handled—firmly not over-indulgently—almost certainly within the first three months your baby will outgrow the need and will then sleep for something like eight hours.

At that point, of course, there's no chance for him to rouse his brothers and sisters at 2 a.m. and when he does wake up in the early morning, they provide him with companionship.

The baby under six months, however, is going to be hungry; and all the companionship in the world can't compensate for milk for long. So even though it's only 6 o'clock on a Sunday morning, if the baby's grizzling I would strongly recommend you get up and feed and change him, and then you can go back to bed with a clear conscience. Any experienced mother will tell you that this is vastly preferable to lying listening to those grizzles become cries and continually hoping he will drop off to sleep again—which he almost never does.

If the older brothers and sisters are early-risers, and you like a lie-in, you have a problem. You could try putting them to bed later at night so that they might sleep longer. If this doesn't work I'm afraid you'll just have to get up early too. It's one of the prices you pay for being a parent.

Using a traditional carry-cot for a new baby to sleep in is

not ideal, because it has high opaque sides. Terribly dull in there with nothing to look at but the ceiling—especially if you can *hear* big sister but you can't see her. Now, I realise this is mainly a matter of economics and that you may very well need the carry-cot for other purposes—for travelling and for carting up and downstairs without the aid of a squad of large men—but if you do have a fond Grandma who wants to present you with a cradle as well, let her. I've seen some excellent wooden rocking ones imported from abroad (about the £10 mark) which have barred sides like the standard dropside cot.

By the way, although the dropside cot is so useful for the older baby and young toddler, it is not a good place to put a new baby. For him, it's rather like trying to sleep in the middle of the Albert Hall when the Albert Hall is empty, if you can imagine anything like that.

Transfer him into a dropside cot when he outgrows his carry-cot (around five months) or wooden cradle (around nine months) and feels cramped, or when he can sit himself up and it becomes dangerous for him to sleep in something with low sides.

If an older child has to be moved out of the dropside cot in order to make room for the baby, this move should be done before the baby actually needs the cot. The move need not be before the baby comes at all, but it should be made as a promotion from the older child's point of view, not as a sign of being thrown out of his cot to make room for the newcomer. To present a bed to a toddler of two-and-a-half or three, and tell him he has now graduated to a bed like the other adults in the family, leaving the cot empty for say two months before moving the baby into it, is good. But to take a toddler out of his cot because the baby needs it and to plonk him in a bed is liable to cause considerable resentment, and who can blame him? I wouldn't take kindly to being turned out of my bed for someone else; would you?

Eventually you'll arrive at a situation where your last child is in the dropside cot and you've no more babies to move into it. What's more, you've run out of single divans. Sorry, but the youngest can't sleep in a cot until he leaves home at twenty or so; you'll have to buy him a bed sooner or later. And the sooner you buy it, the more use he'll have out of it—at least, that's one way of looking at it !

So when he gets cross about being caged in a cot, and when he can not only undo the metal fastenings but he can also cope with the string you tie round them to keep them up, and get himself out, let him sleep in a bed. Don't indulge that maternal need of yours to keep him a baby, because he's your last baby. That's not fair. And don't fuss that 'he'll fall out of a bed and hurt himself'. Honestly, he won't. When you come to think about it, no magic magnetic bonds keep *us* in bed, simply the subconscious knowledge that there's nothing but space on our left. It works the same for children. Occasionally they do fall out, which is why—if you have lino or wooden floorboards—it's not a bad idea to have a rug for them to land on. But they seldom really hurt themselves. If you're really worried, though —so much so that you have to pop upstairs every half-hour to check he's still tucked up—put two chair-backs at the head end.

I've learnt the hard way that it's no good deciding 'at two and a half I shall put him in a bed'. Children vary as much in this as anything else. For instance, it's pretty silly his having learnt to use a pot on his own if he can't get himself out of his cot to do so. And if he *can* get himself out, then it's far safer to be a hop from the ground than a jump, isn't it?

In the case of my own youngest, he learnt to 'escape' long before I was aware of it. Each afternoon I put Nicholas in his cot for his afternoon rest, and ten minutes later I'd find him curled up beside it on the floor. Now, this cot had no ordinary catch; it had been specially carved by an Indian carpenter for the child of one of the viceroys in the late nineteenth century, no less, and it was mighty foolproof. (Nicholas, of course, only acquired the cot fourth-hand.) The cot was always still securely fastened. After a week of this, I began to suspect I was suffer- ing hallucinations, that I was in fact putting my child to sleep on the floor ! Then came the day of the mighty thump followed by loud Nicholas-type screams. He'd missed his footing on the cot-rail and fallen, my four-year-old informed me blithely. I got the message. Nicholas went into a bed, and the cot with the illustrious past was given away.

Now let's consider where to put the baby—and here we are speaking of the stay-put baby, probably under the age of eight months—during the day.

Whenever possible, in the garden in his pram or carry-cot-on-wheels. Sleeping out of doors is healthy and even the youngest baby enjoys it. But the old idea of 'put him out in all weathers; it'll make him hardy' has gone. It is downright dangerous for him to be outside during fog, on nasty damp days or when the temperature drops towards freezing. But on all other occasions the fresh air will do him good.

If you live upstairs in a flat and don't like to leave your baby down in front of the house, it is a good tip to have a solid table near a wide open window and leave the cot on this for most of the day. He will get just as much air—and without being disturbed by well-meaning old ladies. He can also be heard easily if he cries. The open window, one or more storeys up, is strictly for the new baby, of course. Once he is at all mobile, take him right away.

After the first few weeks, a daily trip to the park or nearest green area will do both of you a lot of good. But 'fresh air' should not mean lying in a howling gale or even a little draught!

It is a fact that even the youngest babies get bored. This does not mean that you need a nanny who sits all day entertaining the baby; nor do you have to sit for hours making cooing noises or waving coloured rattles in his face. But it is infinitely preferable for him if you can organise his daily routine so that he is wherever the rest of the family happens to be. If his older brothers and sisters are, for instance, doing homework, there is no reason why he can't lie in his carry-cot in the room where they're working because the normal, ordinary noises of two or three lively children are, to him, a stimulus. The odd word thrown in his direction, the odd person who waves at him or smiles as he runs past is enough to keep your baby happy, amused and interested.

If there are no older children, let him be where you are—in the bedroom which you're cleaning, in the living-room while you are dressmaking; let him be in the kitchen, if possible, while you are preparing meals.

I'm sure you're panting to say by now : 'But doesn't he need to be able to sleep sometimes?' Yes, of course he does. But don't worry about keeping him in a tomb of silence; it's not particularly good for him. The sort of house where you ring the front-door bell and somebody rushes to the door whispering, 'Ssh, baby . . .' is a house where you're going to have an anxious, over-sensitive child.

Routine household noises—talking, the humming of a vacuum-cleaner, the whirr of a washing-machine, water running—will soon cease to worry the new baby. He will accept them as normal and enjoy them as evidence that people are around. Sudden loud noises, close to his ear, may rouse and irritate him. So latch a banging door and suggest that right beside the cot isn't the perfect place for your nephew to clash his cymbals.

The other noise which is important to babies is music. They're not very discriminating—any old music will do. But a radio in the background will entertain your child and help to develop his sense of rhythm and his love of the noise we call music.

After three months, when he will be awake longer during the day, you'll probably find he gets fed up lying down all the time. So when he's not in his pram, either out in the garden watching the leaves blowing or being wheeled along, a Baby-sitta is very useful. A word of warning, though : do check that it is standing absolutely rigidly and safely before you stand it on a table or a couch—particularly after your baby is four months and can rock sufficiently to turn the Baby-sitta over. In fact, once he's reached that active stage, perhaps it would be better to keep his chair on ground-level. Then, even if he does fall out, it will just be one of those many minor biffs he has to learn to cope with. As you'll gather, a baby in a Sitta does need watching; but he will enjoy it because he can see all round him and can identify where noises come from.

So much for the days. What about the nights? In Britain there is a positive mania for seeing that all young children are in bed by 6 o'clock—so much so that when parents go abroad and see Continental children up and about at nine, they are shocked to put it mildly. Perhaps they don't realise that those children have probably had a midday siesta of three hours.

In the same way, your own child's bedtime depends on whether he's had a sleep in the afternoon. If a four-month-old sleeps soundly from half-past three to quarter-past five, wakes then and has his tea, and at six you tuck him up in his cot, he is likely to protest loudly: for he certainly won't be sleepy. He would probably be much happier lying on a rug watching you and your husband eat your meal, and instead going to bed at seven.

Much the same applies to a two-year-old. If he has an hour's sleep in the afternoon, 6 o'clock is probably too early. I'm not saying he can't be trained at this age to go to sleep at sixish, but equally he will probably wake disagreeably early the following morning. (See page 58.)

Some four- and five-year-olds are perky and bright at eight or later; others are droopy and cross long before. Make bedtime to suit the requirements of your own child, bearing in mind he should have an opportunity for something like eleven or twelve hours' sleep. I would, however, add this: I think all children, certainly under the age of five, should have gone to bed by 8 o'clock—not because there is anything magic about this hour, but because otherwise it cuts down the amount of time Father and Mother have together as husband and wife—whether they want to entertain friends, sit and talk, or just watch television. Even if the television keeps your child quiet and content, this is the period of the day which should be reserved for your husband and yourself, rather than 'the family'.

One final point on this subject: we know ourselves there is all the difference in the world between a lie-down on the sofa in our day-clothes, and going up to proper bed and changing into a nightie or pyjamas. Well, I believe it has the same psychological effect on even a tiny baby. Night-time is not a time to be where the family and activity is; it is a time for silence and deep sleep. And I think it also helps if he physically changes his clothes—out of catsuit and shirt and into stretch-sleeping-suit.

The older child will obviously be changing into pyjamas and going off to his room. But if you've one of the sudden droopers —you know, one minute he's playing 'He' and the next, just as

you've started on your lamb chop, he sinks down on the floor—
it might help if he's already bathed and changed. So then a
quick potty and washing of hands is all that's required before
you can get back to that chop in peace.

During the course of this chapter I've mentioned games and
play several times in passing. Later on I'm going to talk about
play in detail, because it is an important part of a child's life
and not merely a way of keeping him out of your hair . . .

CHAPTER FOUR

'Hasn't He Grown . . . ?'

'HASN'T HE grown . . . ?' say aunts and infrequent visitors maddeningly, peering down at your little girl or boy. It's such an inane observation, since the one thing we can be sure about is that the normal child between nought and five years is developing physically all the time. The rate of this development, however, varies vastly from child to child. That's why I'm going to devote this whole chapter to Physical Development.

Most of you who have read this far will probably have seen booklets and pamphlets informing you that your child will do certain things at certain ages—for example, a child will offer Mother his first smile when he's six weeks old. He will make attempts at crawling somewhere between six and eight months, and so on and so forth.

Having considered very carefully what I know about this professionally, what I've observed from watching my own children, and what I've learnt through talking to other mothers, I've decided such charts merely confuse. They have to generalise, with the result that more children wind up as exceptions than as rules. The charts apply, I think incidentally, to some children; but they don't apply to many.

I know lots of babies who smiled long before they were six weeks old. I also know poor unhappy babies from institutionalised environments where there is not the same feeling of personal security, who didn't smile until long, long after they had passed their six-weeks-from-birth mark. Equally, I know lots of children whose first teeth appeared somewhere between four

and six months—which is earlier than the so-called norm—
and I know lots of children whose dentition started much later.

The danger about these fixed landmarks is that parents
tend to worry if their child, according to the chart, seems to
be retarded in walking or crawling or teething or whatever.
They begin to fear their child is a generally retarded human
being. Well, you fear, he might be . . . And how can you say for
certain he is not, if I steadfastly refuse to give you any yard-
sick with which to compare him?

By observation. If you observe your child and note that he
makes definite responses to stimuli, you have nothing to worry
about. If you suspect his responses are not enough or that he
has made responses regularly before which he no longer makes,
then do not lie in bed worrying about it; do not go around sur-
reptitiously comparing him with every other child you know of
the same age. The right and obvious thing to do is discuss it
with your doctor, because he is the best and only person to give
you advice. Even should you write to me, I couldn't possibly
help because I don't know your child; I've never seen your
child. Your doctor has this advantage and—should he have
to confirm your fears—he is in a position to recommend suitable treatment. But he is much more likely to be able to tell
you that your worry was unfounded.

If by now you're crying out in exasperation for a definite
line on what is a reasonable response, let me tell you that you'll
know instinctively. If your ten-month-old rears up on his fore-
arms and knees with ease but never tries to crawl and you're
saying 'Come on, silly, you can reach your rabbit if you really
want to,' your attitude is calm and happy. Subconsciously you
are aware that there's nothing wrong with his spine, that he'll
crawl when he's good and ready. If, on the other hand, when a
door bangs loudly or you drop a tin tray, your child of over
three months never makes any response at all, you become
anxious and desperate. You start manufacturing all sorts of
sudden loud noises in the faint hope he'll respond to one of
them. This is the kind of situation when you are obviously
seriously concerned, and you ought to consult your doctor to
see whether there is something wrong with your baby's hearing.
In the same way, if he fails to follow the movement of a

coloured rattle with his eyes and you realise he has never really focused on anything, then seek advice.

If you live in a large town, you may well have a clinic with a paediatrician (child specialist) in attendance. That's ideal. Frequently a clinic paediatrician carries out tests automatically throughout your child's early life—bone-structure examination at two months, hearing-test at seven months, and so on. Very reassuring, this, for parents. Only a minority of you, unfortunately, will have this facility; but if you are one of the lucky ones, do take advantage of it.

Even when mothers know their child is not retarded, they still compare him with other children, and worry about his 'failure' to stand or boast about his 'success' in walking. Listening to them, I fear that in this modern age women have developed a new disease—the child as a status-symbol.

I appreciate that especially if you live in an area where there are a lot of young parents, the children are going to be a topic of conversation. And it's awfully tempting to score points off one's neighbours. To throw in, seemingly casually, a 'Samantha can feed herself now,' when you know full well *her child* can't, can pay back all sorts of old scores—like her lawn having flourished when yours remained brown and dead! Conversely, it's hard not to feel a bit ashamed when your child *can't* do any of the brilliant things being done by her child and all the other children around of similar age.

Similar age . . . Let's examine that phrase. A month isn't very much age-difference when you're in your twenties, but it's an awful big gap when you are in the first years of life. So to expect your five-month-old to do the things that wretched neighbour's six-month-old is doing, strikes me as very foolish.

Ah, you whisper, but horror upon horrors, your child is the elder and *still behind* . . . Does it really matter? We are not running a race. I hope our children are not out to win prizes as infant prodigies to bolster our pride. And don't be scared to tell your smug neighbour so if she persists.

The reason I'm so anti this kind of comparing data is because it causes unnecessary worry for you and your child, and it's the wrong kind of competitiveness. You should be helping your child to grow up within his own norm, not within a statistical norm. It's horrible to be continually prodding him beyond his current capabilities, just to keep up with someone else. Incidentally this happens later on with even more disastrous effects, when parents say to their child: 'Why couldn't you have made the football team (or the top of the class in maths)? Look at little Johnny next door. Look how marvellous he is . . .' The one place a child should be able to feel that he's accepted as himself is home; and if even there he's compared unfavourably, his sense of security will be severely undermined. This is equally true of the toddler endeavouring to walk or the small baby who can't quite roll over on his own. In the latter case—as we said in the previous chapter—your attitude is just as harmful as your comments.

I've said you should help your child to develop within his own norm, so we'd better discuss how you can best do this. First of all, how do you know whether you're helping him to do something which *he* is striving to achieve or pushing him into something which he isn't ready for?

That's quite simple. Anything you see your child trying to do, help him to find out how to do it. But don't suddenly decide because it's a fine Tuesday, 'today my child is going to learn to sit up'—and sit him, bolt upright, and then be surprised because he falls over. The sort of thing I mean is, supposing you notice that your child is constantly attempting to raise his head, in order perhaps to see something. Then give him support behind his back to take the strain. A very excellent exercise to teach him to sit up is to have him lying on his back on something soft like the mattress of his cot. Then let him grasp your index fingers with each hand, and simultaneously you grip his wrists which gives additional security, and pull. You'll soon find that *he* will pull, using your hands as sort of parallel bars on which to raise himself. And later when he is ready, this exercise will assist him to sit up on his own.

Of course, you may have a child who resents interference —a go-it-aloner. He'll soon let you know. If, say, when he's four months he's trying to roll over but is hampered by his far leg and you push it up for him, he may go red in the face, clench his fists and shout. Seems he doesn't want your help. All right, retreat and leave him to get on with it. The process of learning does not automatically involve someone teaching. Learning very often means just the patient repetition of fragments of physical activity until one has mastered the complete skill, and a child may find it easier to do certain things without the aid of a skilled adult.

We must remember that primitive people never do any formal teaching and yet their children learn to walk; they learn to sit; they learn to smile; they learn to speak; and they learn many, many more complex physical skills than children who grow up in our civilised society ever learn to do. For instance, they might learn to throw a boomerang, or run forty miles at a session, or handle a lethal scythe. So whilst as responsible parents we want to leave no stone unturned in our efforts to give our children the best chances, there's no point in becoming anxious about it, because they'll all learn these things one day.

I'd like now to talk in detail about some of the major physical skills a child achieves in the first five years of his life. For the purposes of casual reference only—and it goes very much against the grain—I shall divide them very loosely into age-groups.

0 – 5 months

The first responses a baby makes are all essential for survival —he cries because he is hungry. His cry is a noise sent out into space in the hope that food will appear. He soon establishes that if he shouts long enough, it usually does. A baby cries when he has pain because he can't deal with the pain and it may also be a threat to his survival—he can't differentiate whether it is or not. But if he makes enough noise about it, somebody ultimately comes and does something to reduce the pain. He learns to recognise you, Father, and Grandmother if Grandmother lives with you, as friends who can be trusted to attend to his needs.

Later he will smile, not because this is necessary for survival but because he had just learnt to use the muscles of his face in this way. He has watched you do it; he has watched all the people around him, since people hardly ever approach a small baby without smiling at him—it's a natural response to a young one of the species. Soon he will be able to use a smile socially, the way we do : to express conscious or unconscious pleasure at something or seeing somebody.

About this time, too, he will discover how to hold an object —deliberately. The next stage from that, of course, is when he uses not only the muscles of the hand but the muscles of the arm as well to reach for the object and pull it towards him. But to start with, the first fifteen dozen times, he does it not so much because he desperately wants the object as to practise his new skill. Perfecting it involves a constant process of repetition. Unfortunately, in the course of growing up, human beings lose the satisfaction in repeating the same thing over and over again, which is why studying becomes progressively harder as one moves from childhood into adolescence and then into adulthood. A child, anywhere up to the age of ten, loves repetition—all his games are concerned with it. Think of Hopscotch, or the earliest ball games he plays. You roll the ball and he rolls it back; you roll it and he rolls it back. You, the adult, get bored long before he does. He'd go on for hours until he was physically too exhausted to continue. It's just as well, too. Unless, as a baby, he was willing to carry on stretching, grasping and pulling back until he was superb at it, he'd never get to the stage where he could pick up a pencil without consciously thinking : 'See pencil; lift arm; stretch; open hand; clutch; draw back.'

6 – 10 months

We have already covered two of the biggest strides often made during this period—sitting and feeding oneself. The third is crawling, or some version of it like the Russian hop. It's a marvellous skill for a baby to master, because it gives him independent mobility—he can explore; he can touch things previously out of reach. Fascinating for Mother when she's in the room watching and a nightmare when she's out of it, because her child no longer stays on the rug where she puts him; he's off on some journey of his own.

How does a baby learn to crawl? Not by imitation, because the adults in his environment are unlikely to be crawling. Not by your showing him how, because it requires a tremendous co-ordination of muscles to get up on his palms and knees and move. He will probably simply collapse again. No; I think crawling is a case that proves necessity can be the mother of invention. There'll come a day when he is physically strong enough and his desire to grab something beyond his radius is overwhelming. When those two prerequisites come together, he'll crawl.

Of course, many children never crawl. They go straight to walking. But if your child does show a tendency to crawl first, do encourage it because it's mighty good for his back.

Towards the end of this age-group and increasingly in the next, be sure you do not stunt your child's physical development (and to some extent his mental development too) by keeping him in his pram too much. I know it's a convenient, safe place for him to be from your point of view; but bear in mind he cannot possibly learn to roll and crawl and stand so long as he's harnessed in a sitting position. So if when he's not asleep, he's grizzling or staring vacantly into space, fetch him out of his pram and put him on the floor, where he can reach for his world himself.

10 months – 18 months

Perhaps standing tempts even sensible parents to join the 'fine Tuesday' people. They think because their child is coming up for a year it's time he stood. So they stand him on his feet, supporting him under the arms, and then gradually let go. This is bad for physical development; it frustrates the child who obviously isn't ready to stand and it certainly doesn't teach him anything. What you should do is to make sure he has convenient furniture or the rails of his playpen so that he can teach himself to stand. When he wants to, he'll pull himself up and then stand wobbling, clutching on to the piece of furniture or whatever for safety. Encourage him, but let him be.

Long before this stage, you may well have bought him the much talked-about baby bouncer. I know bigger babies do love them and I expect they do help to strengthen their legs. But, please, please, don't leave your child in his bouncer for hours on end so that he's wilting with exhaustion—and I've seen this more than once. 'He's as good as gold in there,' I was told by

one mother. 'And it means I'm free to get on with my jobs . . .'
I turned round, to see her baby, hanging asleep in the bouncer,
like a rag-doll. So to all mothers, may I say: fifteen, twenty
minutes at the most . . .

In the same way I find it surprising to note that people will
take a fourteen- or fifteen-month-old—one adult on either side,
grasping the child's hand firmly—and walk him slowly along
the pavement. I can't think what they are hoping to achieve.
They definitely aren't helping the child to walk. I'm not suggesting that the child may necessarily dislike this activity; he will
probably be far too busy moving his feet to keep up with the
body they are pulling along to examine what he feels about it.

A child who is ready to walk will finally dare to let go of
that piece of furniture he holds when he stands, and grasp
something else in the immediate vicinity. He may or may
not get to it without mishap. He may fall down; he may
cry. The contribution you as a parent should make, if he
does, is to pick him up, dust him down, and take him back to
the piece of furniture where he started—without very much
fuss, without attaching a great deal of importance to the terrible thing that has happened. Do not lift him up to comfort
him and thereby remove him from the opportunity of having
another go at covering that distance. Having failed once, it's
tremendously rewarding for him to succeed at a later attempt.

Now, once he can reasonably steadily move from one piece
of furniture to another, the next time you see him taking off,
kneel down a short distance away, hold out your arms and see
if he will come to Mummy—not be led to Mummy by Daddy,
not be led to Daddy by Mummy, not brought to Granny by
Mummy. But see whether he will walk to the person whose
arms he's trying to reach, by his own efforts. When he wants to
toddle outside, by all means hold his hand—but for reassur-
ance, not for support. If he still needs your support, then it's
back to the furniture with him!

There is also not much point in having him on reins before
he can walk independently, because he then depends on them
for support. Walking reins have their place: for instance, a
child who can walk pretty steadily who is taken on a long train
journey will walk much more happily and much more freely

along long corridors—and, incidentally, it's a useful occupation to overcome boredom—on reins rather than being led by the hand.

When, later, your child insists on walking home from the shops (better this way round, because you can carry the shopping in the push-chair) it's a good idea to let him push it by having him walk between the shafts. This stops the inevitable straying of one pace forward and two elsewhere, and it's less tiring for him if he's something to hold on to.

A word about changing from pram to push-chair. If your child likes to sit up or toddle anyway on such expeditions, you might as well take the lighter means of transport. But do bear in mind when you're out all day long—perhaps for a picnic or at the zoo—in a push-chair your child will have to sit up the entire time and he will probably be worn out hours before the outing's over. How to spoil everybody's day, in one easy lesson. (Of course, if you buy a convertible push-chair in which he can lie down as well, the problem's solved. But this type are usually dearer and not so easily folded away on buses, etc.) So generally speaking, I wouldn't advise putting the big pram in the loft until your child is at least fourteen months. Until then the pram is a safer, more comfortable and warmer carrier for your child. Yes—remember when you do make the transition to push-chair, to wrap him up snugly if it's cold and tuck the blanket round his legs, because he won't be nearly as protected as he was in the pram; better still invest in a quilted chair muff.

Finally, it is in this age-group that you may observe your child is consistently left-handed. He rolls a ball to you with his left hand even when it originally landed nearer his right side; he picks up bricks with his left hand—that sort of thing. Now we all know it is far more convenient to be *right-handed* —in our society tools and so on are designed for right-handed people. And because of this, the previous generation decided that all children should grow up to use their right hands . . . with disastrous results.

For instance, every time a toddler went to throw a ball with his left hand, the parents would first transfer it to his right. Later on they'd insist he hold his pudding spoon in his right hand, in the sincere belief that the child would get used to the feel of it there and stop itching to use his left. More often than not, however, it didn't work out like that. Instead, the child got so frustrated chasing tinned pears around the bowl he wanted to opt out of eating altogether. In the same way that ball-game, which started out as fun, became an endurance test and so he gave up striving to do this difficult thing and sought passive activities which didn't require the use of his hands—left or right—at all. Naturally, all this led to his physical development being needlessly retarded. Later still, some children who were *made* to write right-handed suffered a block, which prevented them from being able to read words —the medical term for this disability is 'dyslexia'.

Now, having terrified you out of forcing your left-handed child to be right-handed, I can safely add that you may encourage him to be ambidextrous—both-handed. Sometimes, not always, pass that ball to his right hand. Encourage him occasionally to hold his spoon in his right hand, but when he says 'Can't' in disgust, let him transfer it to his left. Your health visitor or paediatrician will be able to discuss your particular child's 'problem' in detail. She may be able to suggest other ways of helping him to be ambidextrous; she may say you've a true left-hander—let him be.

Accept that he's just quaint that way—I know; I'm quaint that way myself !

6 months – 2 years

TEETHING

There are wide variations of response to the undoubtedly uncomfortable process of the teeth appearing. Some children seem to go through this without any noticeable discomfort, other children have short periods of acute pain just while the particular tooth is being cut, but there are children who scream night after night for weeks on end while their poor parents walk up and down with them in an effort to offer some sort of comfort.

For those of you whose children haven't reached the dentition stage yet, let me say the number of children in this final group is comparatively small. It is not by any means inevitable that you will spend weeks without a proper night's sleep. It is only fair to add that a contented baby who's had correct feeding, no serious illness, and a stable home—and therefore emotional security—tends to react better to the discomfort of teething than a child whose first few months have been physically and emotionally less happy.

And even if you do have a bad teether, you can do more constructive things for him than walk the floor. There are various pleasantly flavoured solutions on the market which can be rubbed on to the sore gum to anaesthetise it mildly. I've heard certain authorities say crushingly that these solutions and jellies are of no medicinal value. That I can't say; I'm not a chemist. But I do know that babies like the taste; they also recognise that Mother is doing something to bring comfort rather than just frantically sobbing with them—an action guaranteed to persuade any sufferer he's beyond hope!

You've doubtless also heard of teething-rings. These are for the baby to chew on—rather as the teething puppy uses a chair-leg. They are generally made of plastic, which from time to time can be sterilised in Milton, but in fact any hard, smooth material would serve. Believe it or not, my mother-in-law gave her children her solid gold bracelet to bite—it still bears the tooth-marks to prove it! But I fancy the common or garden variety in plastic are just as satisfactory to babies.

How about a teething-rusk to chew on? Well, I have clear memories of what must have been a hundredweight of half-chewed bits of soggy rusks which I have swept up from the carpet and dug out of the corners of armchairs, so I have serious doubts about their value. But if you find your child likes something of the sort, then I'd advise a piece of bread baked to crispness in the oven, which won't fill him up to the same extent and won't be another sweet thing in his diet.

If all this treatment isn't sufficient, consult your doctor. He may think it necessary to prescribe a sedative, especially if your baby's discomfort is robbing you and your husband also of much-needed sleep. Oh dear—in case you're confused, *the sedative is for your baby*. I'm not suggesting you should leave him lying screaming with pain while you try to continue sleeping. For one thing no natural mother could relax under such circumstances, and for another the poor child next door would feel abandoned, too, in his misery. If on the odd night he does need you, then you'll both be far better off together.

In conclusion I must warn you that there can be side effects to dentition: your baby's digestion may be upset; he may develop nappy rash; he may even have bouts of vomiting, ear-ache or nasal infection—especially when the back teeth emerge. Though you should be on the look-out for these, I sincerely hope that your child—and consequently you—will be one of the lucky ones to whom growing a tooth is no worse than grow-ing finger-nails.

0 – 3 years

TALKING

Talking is originally a physical skill—that of reproducing a sound; only later does it become the mental skill of communi-cation. A minority reach both stages together. Having been silent to the age of three, they suddenly speak in whole sen-tences. But this is very rare, and most children utter little sounds from a few weeks old. Over the months these sounds become speech patterns—'la-da-da-na' sort of thing—until finally a word is pronounced. A child generally starts with a familiar word which is easy to pronounce. In the case of my own eldest, it was often 'Mummy'.

When Tina was nine months we were staying on holiday with some friends in Kent, and they had a dog—just an ordinary nice mongrel dog. It was a lovely summer, for once, and I used to feed her in her baby chair out in the garden. Now, anything she didn't finish, the dog was always ready and willing to do so for her. In fact it got to the point when we automatically put a bowl out next to Tina's chair and the dog would sit there wagging her tail waiting for the titbits. The dog's name was Dusty, and my cry of 'Dusty! Dusty! Come, Dusty!' used to be a ritual before each of Tina's meals. Then one day she beat me to it, and cried: 'Dutty! Dutty, Dutty!'

It's a thrilling moment for every mother. It's also very quaint that children say 'Dutty' instead of 'Dusty' or 'foobah' instead of 'sugar'; it's tempting for you to start saying 'foobah' your-self. One little indulgence is all right. But keep it at that. The object is for your child to learn your language, not the other way round.

Although I can sincerely claim I have never compared my children's physical development with other children's, perhaps unconsciously I've fallen into the trap of comparing them with each other. So I was secretly concerned when Merle didn't speak at nine months; she didn't speak at a year; she didn't speak at practically two years.

We talked to her regularly in proper language, which is all any parent can do to teach her child to speak. (Mirrors, candles, fingers against lips—these are for the dumb or retarded child and should be introduced by experts.) Merle, in turn, communicated with all sorts of sounds of her own. We understood what these noises indicated and so there wasn't any practical problem. Then when she reached two, my husband and I had to go away for six weeks and leave her in the care of a nanny. On our return we rang the front-door bell and we heard the patter of Merle's feet coming along the hall. She opened the door and said, quite clearly, 'Hello, Mummy and Daddy.' And, much to my despair, I have to report she's hardly stopped talking since! Seriously, what is interesting is that Merle . . . the late talker . . . is the most articulate of my three children.

You see, she'd needed the impetus of someone who didn't understand her noises to force her to say proper words. But a long separation is a drastic method of getting a child to talk. I'd prefer to use patient waiting. After all, some people find pronunciation more difficult than others. For instance, take the French 'oui' sound. Some students say it right the first time they hear it; others are still getting it wrong after years of listening to Maurice Chevalier and Sacha Distel.

3 – 5 years

The average child learns more new things in his first two years than in the rest of his life. By three, certainly, he has usually mastered the physical skills which are an end in themselves. He can walk and run; he has a full set of milk teeth, and so on. Yet the things he learns after that are just as important, only in a wider sense.

For instance, it is comparatively valueless to learn to kick

a ball. It just might have direct application : one could become
a professional footballer and end up earning an awful lot of
money. But generally speaking, the skill itself is interesting and
useful only if we consider it in the framework of handling our
environment : being able to co-ordinate thought, eye and leg.
In the same way we don't encourage our children to cut up
sticky paper with scissors as the first step to being a designer.
We are teaching them to manipulate a tool—any tool.

Tricycles develop their leg muscles. They might incidentally
teach them road sense for the car they'll have one day but,
having seen the fiendish way most tots career about on their
three-wheelers, I tremble at the very idea !

Don't be perturbed if toys and tools manufactured to suit
the statistically average child within a certain age-range don't
suit your child. He may be too old for it, regardless of what it
says on the box. He may be too young for it, regardless of what
it says on the box. Don't immediately assume the worst. I realise it's daunting for the fond aunt who gave him the gift, but
he simply may not be interested in developing that particular
activity at this time, whether it's fitting shapes into correspond-
ingly-shaped openings, handling paints or finding out how to
fill a bucket with sand and build a castle. He may return to it
later on his own, or he may need the company of other children
to stimulate his desire to acquire that skill.

While we're discussing physical skills, I should say a word
about swimming. You may have seen in the papers over the
last few years that experts have claimed—perhaps with some
justification—that any child can learn to swim before he's two,
that it is valuable to teach him to swim before he's two, even
that it's essential to teach him to swim before he's two !

Well, is there a right age for teaching a child to swim ? My
answer to that is the same as to every similar question in this
chapter—yes, when he's ready. And he can be ready anywhere
from two, given the sort of environment in which swimming is
easily possible. Much, of course, depends on the climate. I can't
think of many parents in Britain, unless they are keen swim-
mers themselves who regularly go to a swimming-pool, who will
have frequent opportunities for teaching a small child to swim.
Standing around in shallow water is a chilly business at the

best of times, and our coastal waters tend to be cold; and our swimming-pools are usually crowded with splashing older children or being used by clubs. If you live in a warm climate, however, and you are certain the child wants to join you in the sea, then by all means try.

A two-year-old who clings fearfully to your neck when *you* are in three feet of water is not ready to swim; but a two-year-old who, safely supported on your arm, is willing to splash in that same water, might be. Many small children under five, you know, are terrified when they first meet the vast expanse of sea. They are genuinely frightened standing in water just over their ankles if it's at all choppy. Yet with great jocularity their fathers march them, struggling, into the sea to paddle. This is no good. The child won't discover 'What huge fun it is'; he will simply grow more petrified as the water grows deeper. Before he can possibly enjoy bathing, it is essential for him to become friendly with this element. The horrible principle that any animal will swim if you throw him in the deep end—and if he doesn't, you're there to rescue him—isn't the method for teaching a child to control water happily. As a rule mothers realise this. But fathers find it undesirable, even effeminate or weak, to accept that their child—especially a son—is scared of water. It's silly, of course; we're all scared of something. But with the right kind of handling—'When you've finished collecting shells, if you fancy joining us down there for a paddle we'd be glad to see you'—this is one fear the child can gradually outgrow. So if you think your husband belongs to that category, you might like to leave this page open where he can see it . . .

Incidentally, when you have got your child to the point where he's prepared to move arms and legs if you support his tummy and he says 'Don't let go; promise you won't let go,' don't you dare break your word even if you're sure he'll actually swim if you do so. That could destroy his confidence in the water for ever. Let him take his time. Once he's eight, his junior school will probably give him formal lessons anyway.

Talking of swimming reminds me to say in conclusion that your child may develop physical skills in all sorts of directions which you don't have. My children, for instance, swim very well; whilst I just about manage to dog-paddle in the shallow end. They also play a good game of tennis, and I don't. Please don't feel resentful because your child can do things better than you. Be glad. One up to him. It is just possible that you may have an infant prodigy with a gift for music which far outweighs anything you've ever dreamed of. Splendid. Although you've nothing to be proud of because it isn't your skill which is wonderful, surely you can be pleased that someone you love can achieve something so fulfilling, even if he does leave you way behind . . .

This is sometimes harder to accept in a mental skill, although the principle's the same. I'm going to deal with mental development in the next chapter.

CHAPTER FIVE

'Isn't He Clever . . . ?'

I'VE SAID I will spend a chapter on mental development and the activity known as play; so here it is. Adults, you know, tend to think of play as something children do because they aren't old enough to work. Yet our division between work and play is an entirely artificial one. Actually every effort which a human being of any age makes could be labelled work. Work doesn't have to be connected with activities for which one gets paid or activities which are necessary for survival or even activities which one doesn't enjoy much—like sewing on a button. It would be absurd to suggest that planting is play but weeding is work; that browsing through the loft on a wet day is play but doing the same thing on a sunny one is work. They are all activity, which the healthy mind and body needs.

A baby is working, and working hard, if he's taking milk from the breast or the bottle. He is working when he's excreting; that effort is visible. He is working when he is sitting on the floor examining the curtain hem. His mind and body are involved when he is finding his toes and grasping with his hands.

It is essential for him to explore and to learn to control his immediate surroundings. This environment should become wider and more complex as he grows older, and providing you don't interrupt and inhibit his 'work' it *will* do. Now, this doesn't mean official licence for a child to do anything at all he pleases. It is a part of the learning process to acknowledge that there are certain things which one can't do and there are certain things which one may not do.

For instance, as a loving parent you will want to stop your child hurting himself; but don't over-protect him. He ought to find out about things which could possibly be dangerous. Supervise what he does, naturally. Of course you mustn't allow him to stick his fingers into a live socket. There it's not a case of 'Well, if it gives him a shock, he'll steer clear of sockets in future.' That shock could be fatal. But on the other hand he must discover that there *are* sockets and why we are protecting him from them. Equally, he will never find out why a knife or scissors could harm him unless he is allowed to use them. Obviously never choose your sharpest steak knives for teaching your child to cut his bread; find a blunt one. But show him the blade; let him know he'd cut himself if he used it wrongly. The same with scissors; let him have his own paper ones; keep your dressmaking shears out of reach.

If we are sensible, we allow our children to use ordinary household implements as part of their play activity, so that they learn how to handle them. Using Mummy's hand-brush to sweep the floor, for instance, is desirable. Hitting yourself on the head with it isn't. But no child will ever appreciate what a brush is for if he's never permitted to touch one.

This applies to climbing stairs, learning how a window opens; he must be taught. We mustn't simply put him into an environment regardless of its hazards and simply let him get on with it—he could fall down those stairs or out of that window. Yet keeping him in as safe an environment as we can devise—a playpen comes to mind—is almost as dangerous. Because one day he's got to come out . . . (Not that I'm against playpens for half-hour stretches. They're ideal while you hang out the washing or change the beds. But never limit your child's horizons by putting him in one constantly.)

When we consider how best to help our children's mental development, we must always remember the old maxim : never to force, never to compete with some other child, never to attempt to make a child do things which we think we used to do at that age; but to go along with the child's own efforts to do what he seems ready to do.

I shall discuss the enormous subject of talking shortly, but there are many many other things your baby absorbs before that, almost without *your* being aware of it. He is learning when simply watching the family: you doing the household chores, Father working with tools, the older children at play—this is all entertainment *and* learning for a baby.

He needs the companionship too. He doesn't need only his physical wants taken care of; companionship is part of what he needs for survival—not just for immediate survival but for the future. And gradually he'll require companionship not just from you and your husband but from a number of people. This, of course, is the great advantage of growing up in a family, because he'll get companionship automatically at different times and in different ways from lots of people. He needs to be played with; he needs to have things to stimulate his interest; he needs to be talked to.

0 – 3 years

TALKING

How do you teach your child to talk? To answer this we have to return to one of the things I said at the beginning of the book about constantly reminding ourselves that we are not dealing with someone of a different species; we are dealing with a human being in miniature, and therefore we must behave as though we were talking to a small human being. The fact that he can't yet make the responses we make, is no reason for not behaving as though he could. Cooing and gooing at a baby may entertain him momentarily but it's condescending and it doesn't stimulate him. Talking to him using ordinary language, not baby talk, will help him to talk clearly later on—and just as important, gets us to think of him as someone we can talk to.

With a new baby we at first talk to him about the immediate activities in which he and ourselves are involved. About eating, for instance, we say: 'Come on. This is breakfast. How about having your breakfast?' After that; 'Now, when we've got you changed, don't you think it's time you had a sleep? Would it be good to have a play—or would you really like to go to your pram straight away?'

I'm all in favour of using 'we' in verbal communication with a small baby—you know: '*We* will do this' and 'Let's play',

rather than saying 'you' the baby and 'I' the adult. Obviously
this doesn't work in every situation. I mean, it's definitely 'you'
and not 'we' who are going into that pram! But broadly
speaking, aim for a friendly, equal relationship.

Pointing to an object and saying its name over and over
again in the hope that your child will suddenly repeat the word
has very little value. Children learn what things are called,
and how to pronounce the names, because they're familiar.
If you always say when you go to a particular cupboard, 'Let's
see what we can find in the cupboard. Let's get out your
blue coat.' Thus he will ultimately say 'cupboard' and 'coat'.
In the same way he will learn to name the parts of his body
quite easily because you are talking about washing his *face* and
drying his *hands* and putting his vest over his *chest,* and so on.
You don't have to intone: 'Eyes. Eyes. Eyes. Say Eyes . . .'

Incidentally, there is an interesting sidelight here on the
question of a *foreign* language. I am sure that most parents—
particularly parents of older children who are taking languages
at school—must be aware of the difficulties of meeting French
or German or Spanish for the first time at thirteen. Of course
it's difficult. Thirteen is the wrong age at which to begin.

The right age to learn any language—the native tongue of
the country in which the child lives or a language spoken
fluently by one or both parents or his playmates or the *au pair*
—is when he is learning to speak his first language. It has been
demonstrated over and over again that many children can
learn to speak two or three languages simultaneously before
the age of two. Yes, they do mix up the words and use the verbs
in French and the nouns in English; but they sort out the various languages pretty quickly. Admittedly, they won't learn the
grammar; but you are not teaching your baby or toddler the
grammar of his own language either. Firstly, he learns to say
words; then he learns to make sentences in imitation of the way
you speak; it's many years later before he understands subject
and indirect object. Well, the same applies with a foreign
language. So if you want your child to be bilingual, even multi-
lingual, the time to start to speak it to him is from earliest babyhood—songs, poems, the ordinary communication about
food and nappies and going to bed and saying good night;

about Teddy bears and flowers and birds pictured on the wall.

I myself learnt to speak a second language in a fortnight when I was three. Unfortunately, as I had to do this because I was staying in a country where no one spoke my own language, I promptly forgot my original tongue. Then when I saw my father again, for a while I couldn't talk to him! Drastic, all this, but it does prove my point.

By the way, do bear in mind that you can forget a language faster than you can learn . . . *unless you use it constantly*. Many a mother who passed O-level French can now remember only *'La plume de ma tante'*, which is little use to man or beast.

3 – 5 years

A question which worries parents is whether their child will speak 'B.B.C. English' or whether he will pick up the local accent. (If you're not one of these parents, if accent doesn't bother you—perhaps because you don't speak B.B.C. English yourself and yet have managed to get on all right; you've made a nice stable home and you're rearing a family well—then skip this page, and good for you.)

But for the rest let me say it is undoubtedly a great asset later on to be able to speak in B.B.C. English; it is, however, almost impossible for a child to grow up in an area where a local dialect is strong without his being able to speak that dialect fluently. We must face the fact that ideally our children should be bilingual in their own native language. For the sake of their social relations with other children—and this is important; let us not consider it less important—they should be able to speak the local prevalent dialect, and for the sake of their future they should be able to speak B.B.C. English. So what do you do?

I suggest you do nothing directly. If you dare at your peril correct your child when he comes in with some choice phrase picked up from a chum, then you have hammered that phrase in for ever. He can use it as a weapon; he's bound to use it on all occasions when you want him to speak, 'nicely'.

If you constantly correct his pronunciation, the same thing will happen: you will make him not bilingual, but single lingual—and it will be the one you don't want!

The thing to do is to maintain your standard of speech at

home, and he will automatically learn to do so too, providing you have a good relationship with him. The only reason why children from 'nice' homes speak badly is because they were, consciously to begin with and then unconsciously resisting their parents during the period in which their speech patterns were formed. In other words, if you correct your child and make him mind his manners when he's speaking, you will achieve the exact opposite result. If you merely maintain your own standard of speech at home, you will find he will soon, all by himself, make a sharp division and speak with you as you speak, and with his friends as he finds best in order to survive as a member of the tribe rather than an outsider. It is unfair to expect him to do more. So there's no need to correct pronunciation; on the contrary, it is undesirable.

What is desirable is to correct grammar, and how to do this for the under-five is perhaps worth mentioning also.

If your child comes in bursting to tell you something—it may be trivial to you but still vital in his eyes—and all his words jumble up, and the verbs and nouns go into the wrong places and he says 'me' when it should be 'mine', don't correct him in the middle. Don't cut off his flow of speech. Let him express himself as he will, to get the story out, so that its full colour content is not undermined by your constant, patient, 'No, dear, not that way,' so that he has to go back and repeat it. That's a good way to make him inarticulate in maturity.

But after he has told you the story, in the course of discussing it, you should use the right phrases. Try as little as possible to do this on a *correction* basis but rather on a *correct* basis. If you virtually re-tell the story to him properly in conversation, he will learn to express himself grammatically. And in the meantime you won't have made him self-conscious and frustrated.

I wish more teachers realised this. How often they stifle imagination and enthusiasm due to their anxiety that their pupils should use the right past participle or whatever. I remember that my daughter Merle, admittedly when she was much older than the children we're discussing in this book, once wrote a very remarkable essay. The subject was Law and Order, and she'd chosen a fascinating incident from the Second World War. Her essay was vivid; it was alive; it flowed.

Yet the English mistress's only comment was the old one of 'Punctuation!' So dampening, so discouraging . . .

To sum up 'your child and speech'. Obviously as his awareness of his surroundings increases, so he will be able to express this increased awareness in words, and you must be ready and willing to address him with an enriched vocabulary. Don't be afraid of using words he won't understand. Quite the reverse—*do*. He will learn more words more quickly if you are in the habit of using a fairly extensive vocabulary.

Having discussed the development of speech, we must also realise that talking is *verbal* communication. But it is not enough just to be able to verbalise a need like 'More milk, please'. What enriches life is the ability to verbalise ideas, thus sharing them with others. The importance of play does not lie only in its helping a child to develop muscular skills and understand the world about him, but equally in the stimulus it provides for his ideas.

Although there are many theories about why children play, and especially why they play certain games, I feel that working out the underlying motivation at the deepest level lies in the territory of child psychology and not in that of parenthood. I think it is sufficient to say here that fundamentally children play because it is natural for a normal, healthy being to engage in activities which use his brain and/or body, rather than lying down like a vegetable all day. Unless there is a real emotional disturbance—in which case play becomes something different —or unless the child is urged to do things in the sacred name of play which he doesn't like doing (for instance, being made to kick a ball), he will enjoy it. It should go without saying that you don't force your unsporty son to be a cricketer or your restless daughter to sew. As we said earlier : have the stimuli available, but don't press them. How would you like to be *ordered* to act St. Joan for the local amateur production or play hockey for the county? Wouldn't it put you off for life?

As a matter of fact it's very hard to persuade a small child to do something which doesn't appeal to him. I know a number of children under five who love music and play beautifully in percussion bands at nursery school. But however much one might have guitars, drums, triangles, recorders—you name it

—available, the child who is not interested in making music will not avail himself of these opportunities, at least at that particular time. As we said in the previous chapter, very often a toy marked for your child's age-group will be rejected then but dug out later.

I can give you an actual example of this. My son had a building construction set, a simple one, as a present when he was four. He was totally disinterested. Oh yes, he threw the bits around, he lost most of them, but he made no attempt to construct anything that resembled the superb coloured sheet of instructions. I tried to work on it with him. No. He did all sorts of other things with the pieces—arranged them according to colours, shuffled them, but not what the kit was intended for. When he was about eight, in a friend's house he saw the identical kit belonging to a younger child. He was fascinated by it and accused me of never having provided him with one! He refused to believe he'd had the very same thing four years earlier...

So don't assume because your child rejects building things when he's four, he will never be interested in it. From time to time see that the stimulus to make something is proffered. The second thing to say is: don't consider your child's toys to be your property; they're not. They're his, and if he doesn't want to play, then he doesn't want to play. If he doesn't want to use them the way the manufacturers think they should be used or the way you think they should be used, it is his right. This does not mean that you should permit your child to damage and break toys at will just because he's the owner. Destructiveness for its own sake is irresponsible and self-indulgent and therefore bad for his character.

This also applies to things which are not strictly toys: like pencils, crayons, paints, paper, blackboards. If he wants to play trains with them instead of using them for drawing, fair enough. But he should not be allowed to discard them in the middle of the floor to be trodden on and ruined.

I have come to the reluctant conclusion in the course of writing *The New Childhood* and talking to parents who have expressed a wish for such a book, that to most of them the question of play-materials and toys is a very real problem. It's not merely a matter of money but of knowing what to buy and where to find it, and what sort of things are suitable at what stage. The various manufacturers of toys don't really help. I suspect they make what they think will appeal to and thus be bought by adults.

We as parents do know, though, often from our own memories of childhood, that many bought toys are of little, if any, interest when one is small. Many toys break disappointingly when a sturdy toddler drops them, or they are for *looking at* not for *doing things with*. It is the latter activity which is the prime requisite of any play-material, toy, game—call it by whatever fancy name you will. Toys are not things to keep our children quiet; they are the tools of learning about the world and of learning how to express ideas resulting from such learning. Books for reading to young children also come under this heading.

I can only give suggestions and sketch in possibilities of what is suitable at what approximate age. You the parents must choose what to buy, make, borrow (in the case of large toys like a swing or climbing-frame). A lot will depend on how handy Mother and Father are with tools, paint-brush and needle. Don't hesitate to beg for empty cartons, tins, etc., from shops—they are often only too glad to give away what would otherwise clutter up storage-space. Neighbours and friends are also often glad to get rid of what they call rubbish and what your child would enjoy investigating. Lots of money is not a necessity when trying to supply your child with toys which are fun to explore.

0 – 6 months

I am aware that most parents do the right thing instinctively, simply because they are enjoying the company of their baby. But there are parents who are so busy carrying out the exact instructions on his feeding, his sleep, the hygiene, that they overlook the fact that he is also a person who needs mental stimulus : who needs to learn, who needs time to absorb what he had learnt, and needs to come back to investigate his surroundings in depth over and over again.

A child at this age is interested in the *sensations* which he feels as a result of playing with things. The development of *sensory* awareness of different substances is very important and enjoyable.

PICTURES—Pictures on the wall in the room where he sleeps, pleasant pictures of animals, real or imaginary, are an excellent idea. They give him something interesting to look at rather than just a plain painted wall. (Look out for colourful nursery wall-papers as an alternative.)

MOBILES—These can be bought, or simply made by stringing very light things which are brightly coloured and perhaps shiny, which move in any slight current of air. String milk-bottle tops, lightly-crushed coloured tissue-paper, cut up drink-ing-straws, small balls of foil, on a piece of thin cord and sus-pend vertically in front of the window.

RATTLES—Using stout nylon-cord, string together eight to twelve old-fashioned key-rings (1″ in diameter). A different rattle—because it's a different shape and makes a different sound—can be made by stringing together all the old keys you never use. *Note:* wash these well before use and wash again at intervals. At first suspend these rattles horizontally a good dis-tance from Baby's crib, and *you* give them the odd push to make them ring. At four months and upwards *he* will want to play with them himself, and they will be chewed, thrown on the floor and generally fully investigated.

The hanging fluffy duck which is suspended from the top of the pram-hood and the pram beads which go across the hood lower down are both dull and too close to his eyes.

SAFE, HOLDABLE OBJECTS—Serviette-rings, empty adhesive-tape rolls, empty light-bulb cartons, Mother's silver bracelet, a tea-spoon, the cardboard cylinder from a toilet roll, an empty tea-packet, etc. Put any one of these into his hand and leave him to experience it. It will fall out of his hand after a few seconds because his attention-span is very short. Repeat the operation, giving the object to him several times. After a few days, change the rules of the game. Place the same object just within his reach and if he is ready to play the more advanced version (from about three-and-a-half months onwards), he will pick the object up himself. It will still drop out of his hand after a few seconds. REPEAT. REPEAT. REPEAT.

'Toys' are not the only thing which will amuse a baby and enrich his experience. He likes kicking without a nappy on the floor; his own fingers and toes make fascinating playmates; being gently splashed in the bath is pleasurable, and later splashing himself in the bath. The rocking movements of his cradle, the pram or the car. Watching the play of light and the movement of leaves. And all the games which mothers have played with their children from time immemorial which contain the element of repetition.

Bouncing Baby on a knee; singing nursery rhymes to him; reach and withdraw games, which babies learn to play very easily from about four to five months where you reach out a finger and wait for Baby to grasp it. You then withdraw the finger and wait for Baby's hand to come forward to reach for your finger again. And when he does, you take it away again. A similar version of this is pulling a long pram rattle up, and Baby pulling it down. You pull it up; he pulls it down . . . I know these games are not madly exciting for you, but your baby loves them. They also teach him what response you are expecting, and that is something which we all have to learn. In all sorts of everyday situations we have to know what response someone is expecting from us; so the sooner your baby can start to anticipate this, the better.

6 months – 1 year

Now your child will begin to reach out deliberately to extend his discovery instead of merely accepting the little world that closely surrounds him. He will also begin to communicate, not only about a need but merely because he wishes to form a relationship actively.

THROWING OUT OF THE PRAM GAME—He will throw things out of his pram and, as soon as you've picked them up and given them back to him, out they go again. He hasn't dropped the golliwog or whatever; he's thrown it on the ground quite deliberately in the hope that somebody, probably yourself, will say: 'Ah—telephone-call from Baby in pram.' So the somebody picks up Golly and is supposed to stay there and pick him up again and again and again. I know it's arduous and a bore for an adult. I've done it for many weary hours for many children including my own three, and after five minutes or so, you will probably have to say; 'Well, there you are. This is the last time. I can't go on playing with you any more. I've the dinner to cook.' But for a while do accept this sort of activity as being an attempt at communicating on the part of your baby.

RHYTHMIC MUSIC—to bounce to on Mother's knee or to dance with in Mother's arms.

BENDY TOYS—Choose friendly-looking animals from the display on the toyshop counter (young children get frightened of fierce-looking wolves). Their bendability is useful in developing manipulative skills. But watch he doesn't try to bend the kitten's legs in the same way!

STUFFED ANIMALS—They can be bought or homemade, but they should be small (12″ to 15″ tall). They will probably not be *played with* but they will provide company in his cot.

SOUND TINS—Collect different small tins like tobacco-tins, fill them with different things—some with sand, gravel, dried peas, old buttons, old half-pennies. Seal the tins well by covering the edge with zinc-oxide plaster and paint with non-toxic paints in different colours. These are 'educational' because your child will learn to distinguish the various sounds they make and he will also learn gradually to pile them up.

DRUM—Don't buy *tin* drums because their sound is poor and will be bad for developing his musical ear. You'd do better simply to give him your aluminium saucepan and a wooden spoon. But best of all use an open-ended cylinder (made from a tin which has had its ends removed with one of the safety can-openers), and stretch rubber sheeting from an inner tube over the ends.

BELLS—The Indian brass bell is a favourite. Indiacraft shops, among others, sell all kinds of bells, and half a dozen bells attached to a circle of tape is more fun because it gives different notes. Another bell toy can be made by using a 4″ piece of bamboo rod and threading 12″ of window-blind cord through it to form a hoop. Now attach four to six different small bells to the cord and stitch on firmly.

TUG OF WAR—His old key-ring rattle makes a great toy for playing Tug of War, which helps to develop muscles and is enjoyable.

CARTONS—three of four identical corn-flakes cartons (miniature or ordinary sized) are among the first 'bricks' a child can easily use.

NESTING BEAKERS—Shop-bought or empty plastic beakers, mousse moulds, etc., which you have around the home, will teach him about the inter-relationship of objects to each other.

BEAN-BAGS FOR TEXTURES, SOUNDS, PILING UP AND THROWING—Make bean-bags (18" × 8") out of lots of different coloured and textured materials. (Look through your scrap-bag for velvet, silk, leatherette, corduroy, etc.) Fill small thick plastic bags with any of the substances in the sound tins or others you can think of, but leave enough space at the top so that the contents remain mobile and make sounds. Then place the plastic bags inside the cloth-bags and sew up firmly.

1 – 2 years

This child with his increasing mobility and increasing desire to communicate will still enjoy the toys he had before, but the gradual introduction of some new ones will help his development.

One of his favourite activities will be the GIVE AND TAKE GAME. All through the day he will like giving you an object and having you give it back to him; then giving it to you again and having it given back and so on. The object may be a rattle, a woolly bear or something small he's found on the floor : like a piece of fluff or a scrap of paper. This is *non-verbal communication.* When you send a friend a present for her birthday, you are not, I hope, doing so only because you don't want to offend her or because she'll let you know later that you forgot; you are doing it because you wish to communicate your good wishes with the present. Offering someone a chocolate, a cup of tea or a glass of sherry are also examples of communication on a non-verbal level. Thus the child who is not old enough to communicate verbally, now uses giving and taking games as a method of communication. *Beware:* if your child hands you a tin-tack he's found or some other 'dangerous' object, don't just snatch it away or have hysterics; quietly accept it but replace it with a 'safe' object in order not to interrupt the communication.

PUTTING IN AND TAKING OUT—At first you need only have a shoe-box into which you put a number of safe objects—tea-spoons, screwtop lids, small plastic jars, an old but clean purse (empty!), a smooth arm-bangle, etc. Do this in front of your child, put the lid on the box, and he will enjoy taking the lid off and emptying the box. Repeat over and over again. You will get bored before he does. Later, he will enjoy sample pieces of lino, Formica or even small decorative tiles to 'post' through a slit in the lid of the box. (Make sure the 'posting-hole' is really big enough.)

Around about the age of two years he will be able to 'post' different shapes in different openings.

PAINTING—Yes, it *is* messy, but from about eighteen months onwards it's very valuable. Not with paint, though. Instead use a small blob of chocolate blancmange, rosehip syrup, Ribena or orange-juice (one colour only at first) and just put it on the tray of his high-chair. Don't show him what to do and *don't combine this with his meal*. He will soon find that his fingers make satisfying patterns and the different textures are a useful sensory education and preparation for painting with paints later.

RIDING—A handy-man father can make a satisfactory horse easily. You need a round piece of plywood, 12" in diameter, with four furniture castors fixed at equal distance from the centre. Screw on top a large foam stuffed animal (home-made, covered with old material, roughly similar to a dog or a horse; but it must be sturdy enough to take your child's weight). The whole toy, base and all, should be no more than 15" from the floor. It will aid his walking; and when he is ready to do so, it can then be ridden.

THE MAZE—Your child will also enjoy all the empty egg-boxes, plastic squash bottles, cream jars, yoghurt cartons, and large cardboard boxes from the grocer's to play with. A crawler will love exploring a simple maze built from large empty card-board boxes without lids or bottoms. (You need space for this!) He will enjoy hugely someone crawling in front or behind him, too—splendid entertainment for youthful uncles and aunts and Grannies who come to tea.

MOBILE TOYS—When being asked to suggest presents by

loving relations, make sure that Teddy bears, etc., are not too big for the child. This also applies to mechanical toys like trikes. Raleigh's new trundle trike is an excellent first wheeled *bought* toy once a child is fairly steady on his feet. But always watch for relative size of child to toy.

WATER PLAY—When he is in the bath, offer him a colander, preferably plastic, and an empty plastic squash bottle. The former, of course, is porous; whilst the latter holds water. So not only are these 'toys' fun, but they will teach him something about the different ways in which liquids can be poured.

BUILDING BRICKS—This is the age-group for all variations on bricks. Large wooden blocks, small traditional painted bricks, and towards two different shapes which together form a whole brick.

PULL-ALONG TOYS—Either bought ones or home-made are good. And give him a truck or the 'Mothercare ball-wheel-barrow' to push or pull bricks and other things about in. Pull-along animals, cars, trains, etc., also belong to this age-group, and even after the age of two when your child is walking steadily.

BALL—Look for the new ones with soft indents in foam-rubber. He will only be able to throw it; he hasn't the skill to catch it.

SMALL SHOPPING BASKET for carting things about. He will find his own objects to put in it and carry elsewhere.

HAMMER AND PEGS—Can be bought, or made by a do-it-yourself Dad. It teaches him to create a mechanical effect with a tool.

HOME-MADE JIGSAW PUZZLE—Take a large rectangle (18″ x 2′) of thick cardboard or plywood and cut out of it: a 3″ diameter circle, a square, a rectangle, a regular triangle (all of similar size to the circle). Paint them in bright but different colours with non-toxic paint. Then paint the whole board another colour and leave it up to your child to find out what fits in where.

CHRISTMAS AND BIRTHDAY CARDS in numbers will be enjoyed by most children as something attractive to look at.

PICTURE BOOKS—Stiff board with vivid illustrations of real animals, cars, trees, trains, people—*not* the trendy new books

which look as if an under-five-year-old had painted them!
The story is of no importance, because you won't be reading
it to him at this age anyway. Many children can handle a
book with *paper* pages; if yours owns one, teach him not to
tear it. OLD NEWSPAPER is for that purpose.

THREADING GAME—Brightly-coloured rings to thread on a
rod, or empty toilet-roll cylinders on washing-line.

GLOVE PUPPET—He is not a toy for the child to play with,
but a sort of genie of Mother's. I had one when working on
the children's ward in hospital. He gave out medicines, tucked
small people up for the night and generally dispensed comfort.
By the time I had children of my own, that particular puppet
had gone the way of all good things, but an American friend
managed to get me a glove-puppet Monkey to replace him.
His body was fur and his face and hands were made of a soft
plastic material. Monkey was my most valuable ally. He was
obeyed when the current young one decided to oppose Mother;
he told rhymes, sang songs, fell into the bath, and could sit
on a chest-of-drawers in the children's room to watch over
them, to keep them safe from bad dreams.

His particular value lay in the fact that *I* made him do
things, not *they*. I owned him, but he was a friend to my children. He ended his days in a nursery school where my son had
been a happy pupil for two years; but I have recently bought a
new one, because my granddaughter, who is in this 1 – 2 age-
group, is coming to visit!

Please note that after about fourteen months, your child will
increasingly need someone to play with him rather than playing alone. Try not to be inhibited about singing to him, telling
him rhymes, simple stories, and playing as he plays. Your
housework should be done when and as you can, but it should
not take precedence over the need your child has for your
attention.

2 – 3 years

This is the time when most children enjoy playing *near* other
children, but not *with* them. It seems to be more fun to play
with other children around, although *playing together* will
not take place yet, unless the other child or children are much

older and, as it were, replace an adult playmate. This is also the time when mothers find 'he is constantly under my feet'. Of course he is. He now needs less sleep during the day and he loves doing things when you do them . . . Often with your broom and your saucepan, or one like it. Not miniature household-implements, but yours. (Miniature ones are used much later for conscious make-believe.)

Toys and games should have a definite home—a box, a cupboard, a place where they can be stored conveniently and *where your child can put them away*. If you have chosen as your toy cupboard somewhere which can be reached only by an adult standing on a chair, then you've chosen badly. It must be a cupboard which is easily accessible to your child, because from two (if not earlier) onwards, he will want to choose his own playthings rather than settle for the ones you put out for him. And as soon as he is capable physically of reaching into this cupboard or box to get his toys out, he's also capable of helping you to put them away again.

The over-indulgent mother who feels that what her child does is play and what she does is work, and therefore the work of putting the toys away is something she can undertake (it will only take her a few minutes, she argues), is foolish. She is not training her child correctly, because she is failing to teach him to look after his possessions and to teach him self-discipline.

Many of the toys he had before will still be enjoyed, but he will be able to use them more skilfully.

SAND AND WATER PLAY—If he hasn't had them until now, a sand-box or out-of-doors sand-pit and the possibility of playing with water—not only during his bath—are Musts. Of course you do not organise sand and water play on the living-room-carpet, but in the garden, kitchen, or even his own room if the floor is easily mopped. A zinc bath on bricks to raise it slightly off the floor is an excellent water-container. The water should be about the temperature of his bath, to start with anyway! Provide a collection of funnel, beakers, 'squirty' bottles, spoons, a piece of hose-pipe, a cork, and then leave your child to find whatever else he wants to put into the water. No glass or metal objects please—and don't leave him to play without being

D

within easy sight. Toddlers can fall into a tub of water. . . .

A container similar to the one used for water can be used for
sand. Keep it on the floor and buy well-washed builder's sand
or silver sand. Supply bucket, spade, empty coffee tins, etc,
spoons and scoops, small gardening tools, strainers and sifters,
biscuit cutters, toy cars and trucks. For out-of-doors use—protect your sand container with a fine wire mesh from use by
cats, dogs, and in some cases marauding older children.

Later, the sand and water containers can be side by side :
because *wet* sand has totally new properties and can be util-
ised for building.

MODELLING—a good cheap way of providing plasticine is to
make the following mixture :

Playdough—$\frac{1}{2}$ lb flour
$\frac{1}{4}$ cup of salt
1 tbs cooking-oil
powder-paint (from art shop)
hot water to mix to suitable consistency

Use one colour to begin with and then provide more in a second
colour when he seems to need it.

PAINTING—It is not necessary to let your child draw all over
your beautifully decorated wall in order to develop his artistic
ability. But you should provide somewhere for him to paint to
his heart's content. So for first *finger-painting* efforts, thicken
powder-paint with flour to make it go further and provide
old newspaper as a first 'canvas'.

Later, large sheets of ordinary kitchen paper, available at
any stationer's, make ideal painting paper—the right surface
and cheap to buy. They come in rolls and are sold for lining
drawers and shelves. Pin or nail the paper to a large board—
and a large board means something which is at least 3′ × 2′.
Children find scraps of notepaper inhibiting and prefer a big
'canvas' for their unwieldy scrawls. (If your child proves an
exception here and *prefers* to create miniatures, well then this
is something to recognise and act upon; but as a general rule,
the bigger the better.) Not the finest brushes, please, because his
manual dexterity to handle small things develops much later.
So start with finger-paintings, and when he is almost three
introduce him to painting with large brushes.

Always display your child's artistic efforts somewhere. There is nothing so discouraging as the mother in whose 'nice' house there is no room for 'such rubbish'. BUT don't bore every visitor to death by insisting on the artistic merit of your child's efforts. Loving grandparents will need no persuasion to admire, and you don't need confirmation that your child is another Vermeer or a new Anna Zinkeisen—at least at this stage!

Show approval but not violent praise for what is obviously a first clumsy attempt. Of course you don't say it's poor; but it's almost as disheartening for a child to receive extravagant praise, which is often an unconscious effort to show how superior the adult is. Children have their own standards and they can judge if something is really as good as Mummy says, or on the other hand if it should have gained a little more approval—not admiration—than it did.

Everyone who has created something likes to see it displayed; so choose a wall, preferably in the kitchen, where he can go and look at it, where he knows *you* can see it. This painting or drawing will undoubtedly be followed by another sometime later, and when the replacement arrives, you can take down the original. You don't have to fill all the walls of your house with what is to an adult very often meaningless scribbles. But pin up each one just for a while. After all, it is discouraging and an insult when presented with something to say, 'It's just a piece of paper,' and throw it away. So put it up on the wall; have it there for him and for you—not for the neighbours.

Throughout his life, and not only for his first five years, your child will create various things to give you. However odd these may be, they should be treated as something which you value— not out of proportion, please; not more precious than your diamond ring but precious nevertheless because they are gifts from him. Children can be very perceptive and they quickly realise that their small box is standing on the mantelpiece because you don't quite know what to do with it but haven't the heart to throw it away. Well, try and make use of it—how about a pin-box or a paper-weight? It was obviously intended to be used, and your child will want to see it in use. Don't put it away in a drawer, perhaps to be sentimental over in twenty years' time, when it won't matter any more. *Appreciate it now.*

Moreover, you're setting your child an example. He should learn early on that a present *he* has been given which he's not very keen on should also be treated with some respect for the giver. It's not only a matter of the social form of 'please' and 'thank you' and writing thankyou letters; this must come in too, but later. Long before this, he is capable of making some attempt to let it be seen that a present is being used, being enjoyed.

I have spoken to many married couples who've had this to say: 'My wife's got drawers full of things that I've given her which she's never used. It doesn't give you the heart to choose another present . . .' How sad. The reason for this rejection often lies in early infancy. If a person's gifts to his or her parents have been treated in this way—and it doesn't mean the parents were criminals, only that they didn't understand —then it's small wonder this person never learned the joy in giving and receiving. So the way you react now in regard to your child is important for the whole of his life—his relationships with people long after you have any direct responsibility for him. Again we come back to the point about treating him as you would wish him later to treat others.

PEDAL TOYS—Pedalling (both circular motion on a tricycle and fore and after motion as in a pedal car) are new skills and help him to learn to control a means of transport. The rocking-horse on castors is an exciting toy and much more interesting than the conventional static one.

MODEL CARS—Cars, buses, etc., large and small, should be chosen for sturdiness, not for their value as scale models. And buy friction toys, not clockwork ones.

MEDIUM-SIZED BALL for kicking and throwing, and beginning to learn to catch.

DOLLS—Rag-dolls only at this stage. They are the continuation of the small stuffed companion in the cot, and are valuable for the two to three-year-old because they are representative of a *human* companion. Don't expect your child of this age to play Mothers and Fathers.

MUSIC—This is also the age for the *expression* of music instead of only listening. A tambourine (wood and parchment rather than toy-shop variety) is not very expensive and children enjoy the combined drum/bell effect they create with it. If you are a pianist, try simple nursery rhymes on the piano and leave the tambourine in evidence. If not, try suitable music programmes on the radio or on records, and see what your child will be willing to do.

Maracas, home-made or bought, are a good rhythm instrument; so are bells, two toy bricks banged together, Mexican claves and gongs.

As your child reaches three years or older, he will enjoy singing and will be able to do so with the words sounding clearly. He will particularly like to sing together with other children or with you. (No solo performance for every visitor please—it only makes him self-conscious and is often embarrassing for the visitor.)

I have a treasured memory to this day . . . Whenever I hear the song: *Nick knack paddywack, give a dog* . . . I don't remember the charming children in the film *The Inn of the Sixth Happiness* singing it, but I hear my *own* three-year-old and six-year-old singing to the record while beating a tambourine and ringing a bracelet with small bells sewn on to it.

3 – 5 years

In this age-group I hope your child will attend a play-group or nursery school, and you could do worse than take your cue from the rich play materials offered there.

By and large I would say: watch the directions in which your child's interests develop and supply equipment to assist him to extend. Beware of giving into the whim which makes your child cry for the moon in terms of the toy garage or battery-operated miniature washing-machine. It's often a case of when you've got what you think you want, you don't know what to do with it. In general it is better to give him small things at intervals throughout the year which you are pretty sure will stimulate him, then to save up for that one Big present for Christmas or his birthday.

I could, of course, go on to describe toys and how to make them for pages more. However, I think the ideas already suggested may well have stimulated your imagination, and for further reading I would recommend the following books:

Play With a Purpose For Under-Sevens by E. M. Matterson (Penguin 25p)

The Playgroup Book by Marie Winn & Mary Ann Porcher (Souvenir Press £1.25)

Both give hundreds of ideas, including book-lists of suitable books and exact instructions for the making of toys for children over two-and-a-half.

Let us understand clearly that it would be wrong to attempt to equip children along lines which are not suitable for them. You will see this if I point out to you that if I want to make my child into another Mozart and you want to make your child into another Leonardo da Vinci, but unfortunately, my child is tone deaf and is really only interested in motor cars and your child is colour blind and also only interested in motor cars, then we are going to be in serious trouble!

So you must not try to make your child fit a preconceived pattern. Observe him so that you are constantly ready to assist him, or to seek assistance from an expert, to develop his potential in the direction he has chosen. He might want to carpet-sweep the living-room—that's easy; you can show him how to do that. He might want to know why stones on the beach are a particular shape. If you're a geologist, you're away. If not, you may have to get a book from the library, or consult his nursery school or call in a rock-mad friend.

Of course, he will never get around to asking about cooking if he never sees the kitchen, or about pebbles if he never sees a beach. The stimulus must be available. Heavens, you think, I can't show him the whole world! No; well, to begin with introduce him to the sort of things you yourself like to do. Thus people who read a great deal will quite naturally provide books and read stories to their offspring. Accountants may well play counting games with their children. Painters will draw pictures, etc. It is hardly surprising therefore that often (but let me warn you not always) children show similar talents as their parents.

Many children's games are mimicry of adult activity. This is why little girls play at cooking the dinner or at Mothers and Babies with their dolls, and boys play with hammers or imitate cleaning Daddy's car or—recalling my own son—driving it! The symbolism is very simple : every child, fundamentally, wants to be a grown-up as quickly as possible, and in imagination they are *being* Mother—not just any Mother but you, the mother they know; or they are being Father who puts up shelves around the house and mows the lawn. Incidentally, don't be disturbed if your child identifies his role with that of the opposite sex; it is normal for our age-group.

Don't discourage imaginative play, ever. Even if you are told that something has happened which you know very well hasn't happened in reality, you play along with it.

I'll give you an example . . . Merle, round about the age of two, was ill in bed with mumps on a grey, foggy, dark November day. She was sitting there, looking sick and miserable. Then as I walked past her bed, she suddenly said, quite brightly, 'Mummy, I'm sitting in the sunshine, and I'm playing with the sand.'

And I said : 'How nice. Is the sunshine making you very hot?' (it was obvious she was hot with a temperature). She agreed it was, and I suggested : 'Wouldn't you like to take your woolly off so that you can sit there and enjoy the sun?'

'Oh yes.' So I removed her woollen bed-jacket, which made her feel a little cooler and more comfortable; but more important, she had created a situation in imagination which was enjoyable rather than the miserable situation she was really in. It would have been downright cruel if I hadn't played along and helped her to pretend she *was* sitting in the sun instead of in that hot, feverish bed.

But it doesn't apply only to children who are sick; it applies to any child who is playing an imaginative game. Haven't you heard a boy squatting in a grocer's cardboard box tell you he's driving the fastest car on the track?

If you are asked to join in, you join in. Imagination is beneficial, even, if we must use such a horrible word, therapeutic. The opposite is not. It is against the interests of your child to learn too soon that the magic and glamour with which he can endow the most ordinary situations is on the whole the prerogative of children and that as adults we tend to lose this admirable ability. Don't disillusion his world prematurely. Encour-

age him to believe in 'his car' or 'her sandpit' or fairies or
Santa Claus; it can only make life richer.

When you are playing with your child, help him to take an
active rather than just a passive part. If he's catching a ball,
get him to throw it back to you. Also the story which is acted
out is infinitely more valuable than the one which is merely
read. To start with, of course, you'll have to read it; but overcome any innate dignity and *be* that sheep saying 'Ba-ba-ba'.
We've mentioned several times that children like repetition,
and it's never so obvious as in stories. They ask for the same
one over and over again, until eventually they know every
word of it by heart. Right. That is the point at which the
child becomes the sheep and says the 'bas' and you do all the
other characters. If there is more than one child, the whole
thing becomes almost a play-reading.

All very exciting and hardly conducive to sleep. Whatever
happened to the cosy, nightly bedtime story? In my opinion
it should never have been. These play-readings are not intended for *every* day and certainly not for getting your child
into a drowsy state. And, besides, I'm not saying you should
never read to a quiet attentive child. Heaven help school-
teachers if every single time they tried to instruct, their entire
class couldn't pay attention unless they got up and joined in!

But I *am* saying it is better to have your child or children
told a story *before* they go to bed. It cuts down their ability to
hang on to you for another five sentences or another page or
to the end of the story—and you as an adult have the right
to your own free evening. I'm in favour of giving your child a
picture book to look at or allowing him to have soft toys in his
bed or cot. These are companions; they give a greater feeling of
security which in turn helps him to settle happily to the idea
of being in bed on his own, while you are downstairs. So stories
before bed, please, not *in* bed.

Now, I've gone on a bit about joining in whenever your
child wants you to join in. Naturally, there are going to be
times when you aren't available, and you'll have to say:
'Awfully sorry. Can't possibly today.' Or you may be able to
say: 'I'd like to play with you, but I want to finish this'
(whether it's cleaning, writing a letter or whatever) 'first, so

can I tell you when I'm ready?' And, of course, you'll have to stick to it. You can't then drag out your activity because you didn't really want to play in the first place. There is no reason why you always have to be ready and available; you won't have a life of your own if you are. Your child will latch on to the idea that you're a sort of ever-ready companion, and that he owns you—the kind of situation we talked about at the outset in the Introduction. No, he must learn to play by himself, or with the people or creatures he's invented, without your assistance, and you must learn when you can safely (safely because you don't want to endanger your relationship with your child) and happily (because you respect each other's rights in this matter) say : 'Look, I'll be ready in a little while.'

Phrases like five minutes and ten minutes don't mean anything to a child who can't tell the time. He won't understand whether it's hours or years, but a 'little while' does convey something. So 'I'll be ready in a little while' will usually satisfy him, provided you start on the right foot and haven't previously always dropped everything to come to his bidding. Once more : don't decide one bright Tuesday morning : 'Ah, the regime from now onwards is going to be different. I'm not going to be at your beck and call any more.' This would make him feel cut off and puzzled and he's going to wonder whether he has made you angry because you've never behaved like this before.

As always, it's a question of striking the right balance. If naughtiness can be caused by giving your child too much attention, it can certainly also be caused by the other extreme : ignoring him totally.

You should not expect your child to play contentedly with his toys for hours on end, never needing attention, while you do something complex which requires all your mental concentration. That is the sort of occasion on which you suddenly notice he's gone out of the door and you find him poking in the cupboard where you keep all your cleaning materials (which could be dangerous as well as disastrous for the cleaning materials), or turning on the gas taps, or painting himself with your lipstick. Very often this kind of naughtiness is not just the result of his having investigated what would happen if he did something or other. He knew jolly well if he did this or that outrageous thing, you would have to give him some attenton. What he's indicating is that you've ignored him.

Thinking back, I can sincerely say that, although I have never had a particularly restrictive regime in my house, I have never had disastrous accidents. My house was never arranged to be childproof: the bureau drawers were always full of papers and things, some of them important, some of them probably used envelopes. The cupboards contained saucepans and china. My makeup was available freely on the dressing-table, as it is now. The shelves on which I keep my underwear have a sliding door which even the cat can open with one paw, and therefore the children could have manœuvred easily. Yet never did I come across any of them painting themselves with lipstick or cutting up my slips for bandages, etc.

I can only put this down to the fact that whatever I was doing, I always communicated with them, if only at intervals. A child can happily play next to you while you are busy, if you spare him a word when he asks you to. You can even say, 'Just a minute. Hold on. I'll think about that in a moment,' if you are doing something which requires all your concentration. What you must *not* do is ignore him altogether.

In fairness I should add that the particularly lively-minded child—and this comes somewhere from eighteen months onwards—may well need more than merely the give and take of the ordinary attention you can give him; in other words, he may need the child-orientated environment of play-group or nursery. But I shall talk about this in detail in our final chapter.

A word about the so-called curse of the modern generation: television. Personally I think a proportionate amount of viewing can be very beneficial for your under-five. It can teach him about things beyond your own family's horizons. It will extend his knowledge and stimulate his imagination, and it's a pleasant pastime to amuse him when it's wet or he's convalescing from illness. However, if you let him watch constantly, he'll be in danger of becoming not *square*-eyed but *glassy*-eyed; too passive. After all, it calls for less mental energy to watch a puppet dancing on TV than to look at a picture-book and conjure up the movement for yourself. We, as adults, know . . . Didn't millions more of us watch *The Forsyte Saga* on the Box than would ever consider going to the effort of reading the books! So a limited use of television, please—a tool for learning and a treat—not something to keep your child out of mischief all day long, with the flat-racing, the cookery hints and everything else that's going.

Incidentally, don't forget that censorship is your responsibility, not the television company's. It's up to you to decide what your child should not see and to have the television switched off before that particular programme flashes on to the screen.

You're pretty safe with Children's Television, except that some of the Science Fiction may alarm the very young. Your child will positively look forward to certain programmes like *The Magic Roundabout* just as you look forward to *Softly, Softly* . . . That's understandable. And perhaps it's worth mentioning that you'd be advised occasionally to watch his programmes with him, so that you are able to discuss them. If you don't, you'll lose a point of contact.

A frequent cause of tension between parents and small children (for that matter, parents and older children) is that children are ruthlessly dragged away from games to have a bath, go out for the day, to come in for a meal. There should be a rule in the house—a rule imposed by the parents upon themselves —to give notice to a child that, let us say, in ten minutes he will have to stop playing.

You see, once you regard play as his 'work', you will realise how maddening it is to be expected to abandon your army or your hospital, just when you've got it going, on a count of one. A little warning is a courtesy and it should gain the parent co-operation. For this purpose I'd recommend buying a child a cheap watch as soon as he can tell the time, so that he is able to work out when he must be in and end his game accordingly. But as I've just said, 'ten minutes' doesn't mean much to a child *before* he can tell the time. However, if you're consistent about a ten-minute advance warning system, he'll begin to get the 'feel' of how long he has left. And he'll be more willing to depart from his world for a time and join ours.

CHAPTER SIX

To Love, Honour and *Obey*

THE SUBJECT is discipline. The reason for the necessity of
discipline is that all of us live in relationship to other people
—not only the intimate relatonship of a household but also
the general relationship with close neighbours, with people
who live in our town, with people who live in the same country.
And we have to draw a line between what we want and what it
is fair on others to take.

Thus applying discipline to our children, entails teaching
them to compromise between their own demands and the rights
those who live with them have in any given situation. And
this process begins at the beginning. It doesn't begin suddenly
when a child becomes so unruly that his parents consider him
to be impossible to handle. When a mother moans, 'I can't cope
with him,' it is too late for her to teach him to distinguish between right and wrong; to accept rules for everybody's social
benefit; to instil in him a sense of respect for people and property. So discipline starts when your child's life starts.

0 – 8 months

With the small baby I've been very specific about not letting
him cry needlessly, because if he's crying, he wants something :
food, his nappy changed or perhaps he just wants comforting
companionship. And I'm not going back on that. A baby who
needs something should have that need seen to. But equally
you're allowed a few minutes' grace. You don't have to dash to
him the very second he opens his mouth, leaving the milk boiling over or with your dressing-gown trailing after you. It's good

for him to learn to wait a little, while you get things ready.

But suppose there's nothing to *get* ready? You have just fed him; he's brought up his wind; his nappy is dry; he's snugly and smoothly tucked up; he's not too hot or too cold; he doesn't appear to be lonely or frightened . . . *and it is 2 o'clock in the morning*! He is simply yelling for the sake of it. Well, tell him so. Say firmly: 'There's nothing wrong with you, feller. I'm not going to pick you up, so you might as well go to sleep.'

Better still: use Father's magic touch here. This is often an occasion when *his* No sends the baby off like a lamb whilst yours has no effect whatever. This is because you, due to your intense emotional relationship with the baby, don't quite mean *your* No. Secretly, underneath, you think: 'And if he doesn't go to sleep, I suppose I had better pick him up . . .'

Well, Father doesn't mean that at all! Father means: 'I'm going back to sleep regardless . . . I need my sleep . . . I've got to work tomorrow. So No means no.'

And if it is genuinely a case of the baby just crying for attention and trying it on, he'll recognise he won't win and settle down. But if he sees a loophole in Mother's attitude, he will wriggle through it, in order to get her where he wants her. And the more often you indulge him, the more often he'll expect to be indulged. So don't hesitate to use Father's more-determined No if you don't quite trust yourself to mean yours.

Perhaps the earliest bedtime discipline starts when you first bring the baby home from hospital, and it is very simply this: once he has gone to his cot, and that means after the feed which takes place round about 6 o'clock in the evening, whatever further attention he needs (the next feed, his nappy being changed, later on comfort when he's teething) happens in his bedroom. You never, never bring him downstairs again for any purpose at all. Make an exception if the house is on fire, but that's about the size of the exception! This way your baby won't think about that nice exciting living-room and cry to be taken there. He'll assume that it's not possible after dark; his lot is to stay put.

I have known people who've complained about the difficulties of getting their children to go to bed and stay there. Then, when I've visited them, I've found to my amazement that they have calmly taken their baby or toddler out of his bed at 10 o'clock at night and brought him downstairs to 'meet the guest'. He's petted and made a fuss of and perhaps given a special drink of orange-juice, and then he's expected to go to bed again. And they're surprised that he doesn't want to go! Worse —he asks for the same treatment the next night . . . Well, frankly, I'm only surprised that the parents have any time to themselves at all.

So make two absolutely firm rules—and you and your husband must agree to stick to these come what may—that you will never bring him downstairs after bedtime and that you will never, never, never take him into your bed. Yes: even when he's screaming with pain and you're convinced that extra cuddle and warmth would just send him off. If you weaken once, he'll scream every night until he comes in again. And every woman, and man, has a right to the privacy of their own bed.

As for the very young baby who needs a night feed . . . go into his room and nurse him on a chair. It's far safer (see Chapter Three) and it again avoids bringing him into your bed or out of his own room. Colder? Well, of course his bedroom should be warmed, and he should be wrapped in a shawl, and you should put on dressing-gown and slippers as necessary. But for your future peace, this rigmarole is worth while.

8 months – 2 years

No child is good all the time. If you are expecting your first baby, and you have a rosy romantic dream of a contented gurgling child who grows up into a beautiful adult and then you will be at the wedding with tears in your eyes—forget it. This child doesn't exist, except in your imagination. The nicest child, the most easy-going child, the most loving child will at times be unhappy, tired, frustrated; and quite often you won't even know what he's being frustrated about. It may be connected with something you've done in respect to him that unwittingly you mishandled, or you may have handled the situation admirably but he's misunderstood. It may simply be a case of this older baby clamouring for attention and violating some household rule deliberately to provoke you.

Household rule . . . Have you thought that almost nothing a child does around the house is intrinsically wrong? It depends on the value you attach to what he's touching. I'll give you an example. If you own a very old sofa, a spare one, say, which stands in the hall, you probably don't mind your children playing boats in it, using it as a trampoline, even wheeling their muddy cars across it. But the Louis XIV settee in the living-room, which took you ten years to save for and just as long to find—that's a different story. The children are hardly allowed to look at that without first washing their hands! So you see: climbing on a settee isn't wrong in itself; it depends how the owner regards that particular piece of property.

Please don't imagine I'm advocating a regime where the child may treat his home as he pleases; I'm not. Although a very house-proud mother may well be *too* restrictive to provide a happy, relaxed atmosphere; her child mustn't lean against the window lest his fingers leave a greasy print; he must always have spotless hands when playing on the cream living-room carpet; he mustn't investigate anything that isn't specifically passed to him as a toy in case he harms it. At least she is teaching him discipline as a principle.

Our own children were allowed to do all the above things, but heaven help them if they'd ever torn one of my beloved books or bent a cherished record of my husband's; both were accessible on low shelves. Our children simply learnt there were certain things they mustn't do. I realise it's a considerable test for you as a disciplinarian, but I'm positively in favour of having a tempting 'no' right in the room where he generally plays—the magazine rack, the television knobs (but unplug the TV because its voltage is deadly), a china ash-tray . . . He'll never learn what 'no' means if everything round him is a 'yes'.

So your fourteen-month-old knows he shouldn't touch the papers on your writing desk, but he does so purposely to annoy you.

Provocative behaviour in children from about the age of a year upwards can take all sorts of forms: doing something downright dangerous like reaching for the fire; suddenly out of the blue, hitting or biting you; kicking your favourite chair which he knows full well will damage it; knocking over the milk-jug, and not accidentally, not because he doesn't have the skill to put it down; and a hundred other surefire methods of making you mad.

First of all you say No and you indicate by your tone of voice and your subsequent behaviour that you mean no. Thus long before this 'cross' day, you make sure your child is aware that he's not to touch the fire or kick the chair. And when he starts waving the jug about or slapping you, you say: 'Leave the jug alone, John, or the milk will spill,' or 'Hitting me is rude and it's unkind. Now stop it.' The jolt of No may be sufficient reprimand, but with this age-group I'm afraid it seldom is. The whole point is that they're cross and they want to take it out on you. So I fear he'll be pleased to hear the slap hurt and whack in again, and so on. (In the case of the fire, don't discuss it; distract him with a toy. Don't risk letting him seriously injure himself because he's in a defiant mood).

Well, what do you do when asking him or telling him fails? This is possibly the only book on the care of children produced in the last fifteen years in which the author dares to say that you apply physical punishment. Young children are fundamentally young animals, and I have never yet trained a puppy or a kitten without the occasional punishment smack (and police-dog handlers will back me up here). You've tried being reasonable; you've tried being authoritative, and you've failed . . . *and for the sake of your child's entire future you must not fail*. It is part of your responsibility as a parent to teach him discipline.

So a sharp, definite slap on the hand, the leg, the bottom—whichever was the offending member—and remove him from the opportunity of repeating the incident. (This advice works for older infants too. Pride is very dear to a four-year-old, and he may reckon he's got to have the last biff, if the target's still within reach.) Therefore, take him away from the chair he was kicking or the dining-table with the milk-jug on it, and off into another room. Quite frequently being put to bed will (a) remove him from the scene of his crimes and (b) relieve his tiredness.

Now, just let me stress that physical punishment does not mean beating your child so that he is bruised. It doesn't mean slapping his face, boxing his ears, using a cane, or any one of the terrible things for which parents ultimately, we hope, are sentenced in the Courts. (Incidentally, has it occurred to you that the State applies discipline to those who behave in an undisciplined manner towards their fellow creatures?) But a tap on the bottom, etc., for doing something anti-social—ill-treating you, his brothers and sisters, a friend, an animal or bird, your flowers in the garden—that punishment will be to his advantage.

I'd like to explain in detail what I meant by ' "no" means no'.

Let me warn you that it is usually far, far easier to say 'yes' than 'no'. And some days, often when a child is fed up with his toys, everything seems to be a 'no'. He pulls at a pile of papers on the writing-desk. 'Stop that, Antony.'

He bashes on the french window with a spoon. 'Antony, no.'

He kicks at the gate across the stairs. 'No.'

He goes back to the papers again, and Mother thinks: 'Perhaps it wouldn't matter if I let him play with just that one. After all, it is only a circular, and I've read it . . .' 'All right, Antony, just that one. Oh, if you must—Aunt Amy's letter too, but no more . . .'

I'm willing to bet that at bedtime she'll be gathering up the entire pile of papers, all of which have been screwed up or torn.

And her child has learnt a lesson: Mother doesn't mean 'no'—not if you push her long enough.

And she should have meant no because she needed the gas-bill and the bank-statement intact. If those papers had *all* been old circulars and your child had fancied playing with them, in that instance it would have been kind to have allowed it. But if you're going to say 'yes', you must say 'yes' from the start.

Whenever your child makes a request, I advise you always to consider first whether it is reasonable and you can grant it. I'll give you an example where a mother might be tempted to refuse. A twenty-month-old boys says: 'Jumbo. Want Jumbo.'

'No, not now,' says Mother, because spongy Jumbo is in the cupboard upstairs and she doesn't want to be bothered to fetch it. Child begins to fret, and Mother tries to distract him with other toys. Child gets cross, repeatedly shouting for Jumbo. Mother realises it will take far less of her time and emotional energy to climb those stairs and fish out Jumbo than to play here with her son in an attempt to appease him. So she complies and is rewarded with peace.

But once again Child has learnt a lesson: if you want a thing, keep on whining for it and eventually Mother will give in. And all too soon this principle is extended from a reasonable request to an annoying one, like wanting drinks of water throughout the day, to something intolerable, like picking the heads of the prize begonias in the park.

I was in the baker's the other day when a mother came in with her two-year-old, who was clutching a still-dripping lolly-stick.

'Caikie!' demanded the little girl, pointing to a Viennese pastry.

'No, darling,' said Mother, 'you've just had a lolly, and some chocolate before that.'

'Caikie!' shouted darling.

Mother paid for the bread she'd come in for, and by now her daughter was positively screaming. 'And one of those cream cakes,' Mother added resignedly to the assistant.

I swear to heaven I didn't speak. Something of my shock must have shown in my face, though, because Mother turned to me and said: 'I have to give in to her. If I don't, she screams. She's got a grabbing nature, you see.'

I saw all right. Here was a mother who had never said 'no' and meant it. And she excused her own weakness, her failure, by blaming 'her child's grabbing nature'. I will admit that there are a few children whose inherited genes create a tendency in them to be mean, unstable, violent, etc. But I firmly believe that the vast majority of *selfish, unpleasant, demanding* children would have been perfectly acceptable little people if only their parents had disciplined them correctly. The girl in the baker's had a 'grabbing nature' because she'd been taught that if you demanded loudly enough, you got.

With every child from about sixteen months old, you will have defiance about going to bed. What is wrong with going to bed? Mainly, that he's going there without you. We have to remind ourselves that once, not so long ago, he lived in intimate, continuous contact with you, and now there are increasing periods when he's away from you. Isn't he bound to crave your physical closeness? He also imagines (not so far wrongly) that a lot of exciting things are going to happen the very moment he is sent to bed. Tough. But he needs his sleep and you need your evening.

So do not allow him to prolong the bedtime ritual. As we said in the previous chapter: it's inadvisable to undertake stimulating activities at this juncture, like acting a story. But that's no reason why you shouldn't invent something to make going to bed appear just a little desirable, like seeing how quickly both of you can get there, or having a race from bathroom to bedroom is a useful tool. It is something he can look forward to every night, and it has the sneaky advantage of hurrying him up.

You may well ask why I'm dealing with this under 'Discipline'. As you know, I'm a great believer in avoiding a problem rather than having to solve one later on. And if your child grows up hating or fearing bed, you'll get this sort of dialogue every evening :

> 'Don't want bed.'
> 'Yes, you do; it's bedtime.'
> 'Not !' Tears appearing.
> 'Come along. Good boy . . .'
> 'No !' Going rigid, starting to cry.
> 'Yes.' Taking hand and pulling upstairs.
> 'Hate you. Hate you . . .' Exit screaming child.

Very often the more fatigued the child is, the more difficult he is about bed; but you must start as you mean to go on. If you once stay with him, lie down on his bed next to him until he's asleep, you shouldn't be surprised if when he's eight years old he still expects you to do so. I have known a few mothers in my time whose husbands sat for anything up to three hours every night alone while Mummy was desperately trying (a) to creep away from the bed, and as soon as she succeeded the child would rouse and yell so that she'd rush back to him again, or (b) to keep awake having lain down next to the child! Poor old lonely Dad down there, being denied his right to her companionship. But don't blame the child. This extraordinary state of affairs was started by the adult.

If the child is accustomed from the beginning to being put to bed when it is bedtime with whatever small ritual helps him to be happy, then you won't have any serious trouble. You'll get complaints and pleas. No normal, healthy child *wants* to stop playing and lie down. The only one I ever knew who regularly said: 'I'm tired, Mummy. Can I go to bed?' had recently had a hole in the heart operation. Though your child may not go willingly, he'll go reasonably.

If he feels lonely up there on his own, let a doll or Teddy sleep in the cot with him. If he seeks companionship, a companion would seem to be the logical answer. He may be afraid of the dark, or pretend to be afraid of the dark, in which case I'd suggest a small nightlight—and by that I mean an electric one. Leaving his door open so that he can see the light shining from the hall and hear distant, comforting noises from downstairs will also help.

But there's a difference between granting those sorts of requests and the everlasting 'drink of water' or the father who when he said goodnight to his son also had to kiss seventeen toy animals all round the room! The latter are extreme examples of what not to do: examples of very efficient disciplinary action of child against parent! They frustrate you, and will achieve nothing but harm for your child: for they teach him that *you* have to compromise; he doesn't. If he shouts loudly enough and often enough, he wins. And you should be the winner—not because you are bigger but because you are wiser.

Then just when you think you've got young Timothy to the stage when you can say 'Bedtime in ten minutes,' and he'll groan but start packing cars into garage, he turns round and says: 'Not bedtime!' A nasty shock, this. But eighteen months to two years is a perverse age; they will oppose everything. Whatever you suggest—no, they want to do something else.

A mother may well say to her twenty-one-months old little girl, 'Would you like to put your red dress on?'

'No. Don't want to put my red dress on!' Now, Mother is rather puzzled because she knows her young daughter likes the red dress.

'Which dress would you like to put on?'

In fact the little girl doesn't want to put on any dress, because she's just being contradictory. She is being Mary, Mary, quite contrary. It's a phase. By the time she goes to school, if you've handled it rightly, she'll have outgrown it. If you haven't, she will tell you what dress *you* are going to wear!

So as soon as you recognise that your child has entered the phase of contradicting, don't suggest; tell. 'Today we're going to put on the red dress . . . We are now going out for a walk. The sun is lovely and we're going shopping.' No question of 'would you like to?'. The phase will pass much faster if the child can't play Boss; if he can't dumbfound you by replying: 'No, I don't want to go shopping.' Because that's what he's doing: pitting his will against yours to see who's going to be boss.

And, believe you me, in his heart of hearts he wants *you* to tell *him* what to do. He wants the security of knowing you have the strength to make the decisions, and to find this out he has to test you. So you indicate to him without any clash that you do have the strength. If you don't, you're not fit to be a parent. Sadly, too many children under five have already learnt that their mothers and fathers are not fit to be parents, and that is pathetic because the parent who is weak has experience, and the child who is so much stronger hasn't. The result, of course, is chaos: the child cannot handle himself; he can't teach himself; he can't educate himself. And there is no one to help him.

$2 - 3\frac{1}{2}$ years

By the time your child has passed the two-year mark, his misdemeanours will probably annoy you far more. You're aware he knows perfectly well what he's doing and yet what he does is to defy you. And I talk of a sharp slap! I know it's easy to lose your temper when the little beast tips red paint over your white curtains, or perhaps he has carried on banging a door you've twice asked him to close and, under stress of emotion totally unconnected with the crime—business worries, family problems, your health—you over-punish. That slap becomes an angry wallop. You yell at him and whack, whack, whack.

Then, having done so, having relieved your own feelings, you then naturally think: 'Oh Lord, what have I done! My poor child!' Right—think it; but don't do anything about it, not then. Don't take him into your arms and, as it were, negate by verbal comfort whatever usefulness might have come out of your having indicated your disapproval so violently. Instead, when you feel more reasonable and when the child has calmed down, an apology will suffice. 'Look, I'm sorry I had to hit you so hard, but what you did was rather awful.' The child will remember the smarting bottom and so the effectiveness of your giant-sized punishment won't have been lost for the future; but your apology will assure him that you didn't hurt him because you hate him. Your love is still his. You simply lost your temper. Children have an innate sense of justice. They almost never resent retribution; it is only the unjust punishment that festers. So let him see why he made you cross, and he'll accept philosophically that the extra spank was for choosing a bad moment.

It is generally true to say that any child who has violent emotions will not be helped if we match our emotions to his. I am thinking here particularly of the child who is given to tantrums. Slapping him and shouting at him in the middle of his tantrum is merely going to cause a clash between your temper and his. It isn't an application of discipline. It may be an outlet for you, but that isn't the object, is it?

The correct way to deal with a tantrum is to keep calm and to remove the child from the place where it occurs. Preferably get him alone with you, not surrounded by worried, frightened, perhaps over-indulgent grandparents and friends whose reaction unconsciously encourages a scene. In a quiet atmosphere your child will cool down faster.

I'm not talking through my hat; I *know*. I have a daughter of my own who is given to intense emotions and opinions, and when she was little she suffered—rather the *whole family* suffered—from her violent tantrums. At times she got so pent up with frustration, because the world frequently had the audacity to go its own way instead of hers, that there was sometimes a real danger of her attacking her brother or sister, us, friends, or even doing herself some damage. With all this suppressed emotion bubbling under the surface she was certainly not exactly a pleasant person to have around. I was forever carting her off into empty rooms and talking to her calmly. I got heartily fed up with it.

Then one day I decided to sacrifice a large cushion, the largest we had. It was bright orange and stuffed with foam-rubber chips. She began a tantrum and I took her into her bedroom, gave her the cushion and said : 'Now, I don't care what you do to this, but you do it in here alone. When you feel fit to re-join the human race, you can come out again.' Note I gave her the freedom to decide for herself when she had got over what made her feel so dreadfully tight and furious.

I don't know what she did to the cushion on the first occasion; there was a great deal of noise going on in there, and I kept away. But she reappeared twenty minutes later looking quite different, obviously feeling happier, and joined in with whatever the family were doing. We behaved as though she'd just come in from the garden : no inquests, no scoldings. For the next few years we used the cushion, or I should say *she* used the cushion, because it became a voluntary act, whenever she felt a tantrum coming on. It got to the point where she would say, with barely suppressed tears, 'I'm going to see my hate cushion,' because that became its nickname : the hate cushion.

If you're wondering what on earth she did to it, you'll sympathise with my own curiosity. One day I peeped round the door. She did just about everything you can imagine to her cushion—she bit it; she pummelled it; she kicked it; she threw it; she buried her head in it; she (if you will pardon the symbolism) killed the cushion. But she got rid of that excess of fury.

You may well ask how did I know it would work? Perhaps the simplest answer to that is I am a person of violent emotions myself. There have been many occasions when scrubbing a floor or beating a carpet or savagely brushing the path has been a great relief to my feelings. It used up my angry energy. But I couldn't get a two-and-a-half-year-old to scrub the floor or beat a carpet; so I hit upon the cushion idea. But I knew instinctively that it had to be a private confrontation. She had to be helped to help *herself* control those strong feelings. I feel sure that if one controls a child so that he doesn't show his feelings, one will merely suppress them instead of eradicate them. They'll only come out in some other, probably less desirable, way.

In this age-group also you will get the runaround at bedtime. He's not such a little thing any more; he's not dying to close his eyes. So he looks about and plots ways to summon Mummy. A drink of water is always good for starters. Don't fall for it. He doesn't want a drink, though he may force down the one your pour for him—he wants you upstairs. A neat way of combating the young child who claims to be 'gasping with thirst' is to offer him a drink of water last thing. That way you know any genuine thirst has been satisfied. (The draw-back to this is you may create a wet nappy problem. Choose your lesser evil.)

So drinks are out . . . 'Mummy, I've got a secret to tell you . . .' 'I want to kiss Daddy goodnight . . .' 'Mummy, my—er—er—head hurts . . .' Oh, there are lots of fine reasons for you to go to him, and not one of them is necessary.

Once he's in a bed, of course, he can get out and come down to you. They know how to look very appealing in their nightthings, clutching Teddy and standing in the doorway. Daddy especially may well be seduced by his little girl's smile and cuddle her. On your own heads be it. I strongly advise you to march infant straight upstairs again without so much as a Hello.

In the case of an ordinary healthy child I really cannot think of anything which is liable to happen that would require you to talk to him again before morning—regardless of visitations, calls, demands for this, that or the other.

And don't assume that if you go upstairs because your child has shouted for a drink of water four times and instead of giving him that drink you slap him, you've achieved the right disciplinary measure, for you haven't. Although you've slapped him, you've also made the effort to go upstairs and give him attention, which is what he really wanted, and bad attention is better than no attention at all.

Please notice that earlier I did say *healthy* child. If your child is ill with ear-ache (and you know whether he's malingering or not) or has measles, for instance, then naturally he will need your comforting presence. He may well feel fretful and be unable to sleep because he's uncomfortable and feverish. So when *he* calls or cries, I believe strongly that you should answer. But again you must be careful during his convalescence to withdraw your constant companionship: otherwise you will still be running upstairs perhaps fifteen times a night when he's ten, and you'll be saying: 'You know, he was fine until he was three, but then he got the measles and ever since then he can't sleep and I have to go to him . . .'

The same applies to a child who is mentally disturbed. He wakes screaming with terror from a dream. That is genuine distress. Don't say in this case, 'There's nothing he could possibly want; let's leave him to scream.'

$3\frac{1}{2}$ – 5 years

Most three-year-olds tell whoppers. Now, when we consider lying and what disciplinary action we should take against it, we must clearly differentiate between three things: the child who is creating fantasy, the child who lies to get himself out of possible trouble and the child who is chronically unable to come to terms with reality—and children in that last category, who are in a very small minority, need expert help not punishment.

We have already discussed fantasy in play: the child who makes believe a cardboard box is a racing car. Sometimes they will simply come out with: 'I'm goalie for England.' Don't get all worried your small son is suffering from delusions; he's perfectly aware he's not really. You don't have to point it out. As long as it is tacitly understood by both you and child that this is a tall story, a good story, a bit of fun, a game, play along.

'There now! So why didn't we win the World Cup? Did
you let in too many goals?'

'No. I was at the seaside that day.'

'Oh, that was the day you swam the Channel, was it? Only
I reached France first . . .'

My children and I have told tall stories quite deliberately,
and seen how tall they could get. My middle daughter, the
one with the tantrums and the superb imagination, frequently
shocked ladies on buses by telling them that she was really a
Martian in disguise! For older children there is a game which
they thoroughly enjoy called Cheat, which exploits fibbing for
all it's worth. Personally I don't think it does any harm, providing everyone agrees that *this is a game which the family
are playing for a specific time only*.

So that leaves the middle category: the child who lies to get
himself out of trouble. Heinous crime, you say. Well, you'd
just better be sure he never catches you telling an acquaintance you're so sorry you can't attend the choir afternoon but
you're going out, *when you're not*. 'You *lied*, Mummy,' he'll
say, shattered. Anyway, let's assume that tricky situation won't
happen. First of all you need to be sure that your child *is* lying.
You must learn to understand the tone of his voice, his attitude,
his whole behaviour when accused of telling a lie; so that you
can be sure of the facts. If in doubt, under British justice he's
innocent . . . although he may confess later!

Well, if you can persuade him to admit finally that he com-
mitted the crime, whatever it was, and therefore that he lied
to cover it up, it might just be worth while on this occasion
letting him off the original punishment as a reward for owning up. If he never owns up, but shamelessly continues to
blame his sister, or his playmate or the cat, and you have
proof that he is lying, then give him a double punishment—
half for the crime and half for the lie.

Discipline inevitably involves punishment—for instance, I've
just mentioned a double punishment for lying. But how
should you punish? I've already discussed reprimands for a
first offence and slaps for subsequent offences. Trouble is: it
isn't always convenient to smack your child. A good example of

this is when you're out shopping. You're in a busy street; the child is bored, tired and cross and he provokes you. Apart from not wishing to lose your own composure by having a physical clash with him, it would be unfair on him. Public humiliation involves a loss of face, in his eyes way out of proportion to the size of his crime.

This is also true of a crowded room at home. If Father, Granny and particularly his friends or brothers and sisters are present, it's much better to take your young delinquent away and administer the slap out of sight and earshot.

But going back to the street . . . there you don't have the chance to take him elsewhere, and to hit him two hours afterwards, when you're home again, strikes me as almost sadistic. So what are the alternatives? You can withdraw extra privileges—ice-cream that you were going to buy when you passed the newsagent's, for example. Or a special outing he was looking forward to, like a trip to the coast. But do bear in mind he might not be the only one looking forward to it! And having once said, even in a temper, 'Right. You were naughty; you won't go to the coast on Sunday,' you'll have to stick to it. And even if Sunday is blazing hot and the whole family is itching for that day out, you'll have to settle for a walk in the local park. Much as you realise, 'It was a stupid thing to have said,' if you dare go back on it, your child will know for all time that your threats are empty ones.

For the child in a temper: sitting him somewhere, perhaps still shouting, until you tell him he can get down is a punishment with a calming effect. But you may have to order him back there several times, because *he* must not be allowed to decide when he's served his sentence. On the other hand, don't go away to do the washing and forget all about him! For other children, like my daughter, it works better if you do let her be the judge: 'You stay in your room until *you* think you are capable of coming out.'

But *locking* a child in a room is never, never, never justified. Whatever he's done, this is still his home, not a prison. Withdrawing food is also wrong. The old Victorian 'You go to bed without your supper,' or 'You'll go to bed with a cup of water and a piece of dry bread,' should belong only in fairy tales. Equally, 'I won't love you . . . . If you do that, Mummy can't love you,' is a cruel thing to say to a child. You should love him always, and he should know it . . . even when you have to smack him.

Strangely enough, children are well aware that those who apply discipline correctly do so because they love them. Children know that they need firm handling. Not only do small children know this, but teenagers know it, too. Very often the outrageous things they do are a bid to make their parents care about them enough to say No. One of the saddest comments I heard the other day from a girl was: 'My school aren't exerting sufficient pressure. They're not making me work hard enough.' You see, she knew she was not yet able to apply the required discipline to herself and yet nobody else was prepared to do so for her.

So children accept that they need to be told what to do; they even accept that they need to be punished for failing to do it, and therefore they respect those who apply discipline correctly and have contempt for those who don't. So be a parent your child can love and admire, not despise.

Now, it's not much good one of you being fair and just if the other parent spoils the child at every turn. A united front before the child always, if you expect your punishments to be effective. Of course, you may later, in private calm discussion (not in an accusatory row whose atmosphere permeates the house so that your child knows anyway that you didn't agree about it), state that you didn't think such-and-such a punishment suited the crime. Then you can come to some mutual, satisfactory arrangement for future occasions. But in front of the child you must present an unyielding, shoulder-to-shoulder front line.

You must never allow a situation to arise where your child knows he can play one of you off against the other. As a little girl I discovered only too soon that I could play my mother off against my father and vice versa, and I managed to carve out a pretty cushy life for myself by doing this over many years. In fact, I got them to the point where they unconsciously encouraged me! When I persuaded my father to let me do something which I knew my mother disapproved of, he'd wink and say : 'All right, but don't tell your mother!' The converse was also true. Well, my parents are text-book examples of poor disciplinarians.

On this subject I should also repeat something I said in Chapter Three. It is essential that you carry out punishments yourself. In other words, you don't say : 'You wait till Daddy comes home . . .' How unfair on the whole family to thrust Father into the role of the Big Bad Wolf. It makes him feared, you despised, and the child himself insecure. It is also dangerous to cast policemen as Nasty Men : some day your child might need a policeman's help desperately . . .

In the same way it is very silly to threaten a child with school. 'If you are naughty, I'll send you to school.' If you say that, you cannot be surprised that your five-year-old, when the great moment comes to enter into what should be an exciting adventure, resists with all his might. He'll think you are only pretending school is nice because you used to say it was a punishment.

All parents of under-fives will find the day dawns when they hear their child swear, and they will immediately feel obliged to put a stop to it. You can't stop it by opposing it. Punish your child for swearing and you will have made him swear for ever. No, there is a tried and tested method for curing swearing children, and it's the same method I apply on bumptious adults who insist on hurling obscene language at me. I do nothing; I ignore it. Very soon the swearer gets tired of using his explosive phrases, because I don't seem to notice them or, if I do, they don't seem to shock me. And they were meant to. He'd learnt them specifically for that purpose. So the swearing phase passes with disillusionment.

I carried out this routine with my own three children, one after the other. The end result is that none of my children swears. The only person in our household who still swears is me—probably because years and years ago my ladylike mother was so satisfyingly horrified!

To conclude this chapter may I say that the number of times when you have to apply discipline will largely depend upon your child's temperament and your own, and the extent to which you have a friendly, human relationship rather than a parent-child one. It is generally true that the more you use real consideration and courtesy towards your child in speech and action, the fewer situations will arise which call for firm disciplinary measures.

It is not by chance that I have entitled the chapter 'To Love, Honour and Obey'. Certainly I agree he must learn to obey you. But in turn you should honour him—and that means having respect for his rights and his feelings. And, most important, you should love him at all times, even when he fails and disappoints you.

CHAPTER SEVEN

There *Is* a Substitute for Mum

HEAVEN HELP us, there's got to be. Otherwise you'll be sitting in the desk beside your child when he takes his A-levels . . . 'because', you'll explain to the examiners, 'you see, he's never been without me'! So let's be practical. If he is one day to grow into an independent adult who can mix naturally, then he must be encouraged in infancy to take a few steps away from the apron strings out towards people other than you and his father. True, you, Mother, are the pivot of his existence but, as we said right back in the Introduction, it's not fair on either of you to treat this as a reason for chaining yourselves together.

There are going to be occasions when you simply have to go somewhere and it is physically impossible for him to come too. Take your six-weeks post-natal examination . . . It is likely you will have to return to the maternity hospital for this. A simple six miles in an ambulance when you went in before and a simple six miles in your husband's car when you came out. But this time you've got to make the journey by *public* transport : which involves a walk to the station, three stops on the train and a bus the other end . . . and the only transport you have for Baby is a carriage-built pram. Well, he'll just have to stop behind for a couple of hours.

But the reason for leaving him doesn't have to be as serious as this. You'll be condemning yourself to a grim, grey future if you decide that never again can you and your husband go out in the evenings, never can you browse through London dress shops for a whole afternoon, never ever can you plan anything which doesn't include your child.

Now I'm going to state quite categorically that no small child should ever be left totally alone in the house or flat, even if it is only for a short time; even if he is safely in his play-pen, or strapped into his pram, or asleep in his cot. And so if *you're* not around to take care of him, a baby-sitter must be.

Like everything else we've dealt with in this book the process from total dependence on you in the womb to enjoying a week's holiday staying with someone else has to be *gradual* one. You must not be available every second until he's six months and then when he is fully weaned off the breast, or at eighteen months, because he can then walk on his own, say: 'Right, biologically he's independent of me. Mrs. X can look after him.' If you do, the shock of suddenly finding himself bereft of the figure of love and comfort he knows may have a deep and bitter emotional effect on him. He needs to learn slowly and gently that others can be trusted, and that Mother always comes back to him again.

After all, the daily loss of Father from eight in the morning till six at night, or whatever, is unhappy-making for him; but the fact that Father reappears just before your child goes to bed, reassures him and gradually accustoms him to such a routine. (I am aware that there are many situations where this cannot happen—a husband may well return home long after his child's bedtime, or he may have to be away for weeks on end. I am merely creating the ideal, the aim.) Incidentally, always remember that Father's presence is of almost as much importance as Mother's. This is not said to flatter fathers, but based on fact. It is well known to welfare workers, probation officers and others who are concerned with the care of young people, that the continuous absence of fathers during World War II increased the percentage of teenage offenders, who seemed to need to hit back at the world. Those fathers were in the main absent during babyhood and early infancy, not the later years.

0 – 15 months

We also said in the Introduction that mothers should not forget that they are wives too. Certainly within the first three weeks after Baby is born, it is desirable that one evening is set aside for husband and wife to go out together as man and woman, if only to the pictures or to visit some young friends who haven't any babies of their own.

Now although this may sound heavenly when you arrange it, at the moment of departure you may resist. Don't forget the other half of that umbilical cord was joined to you. It's quite natural that you should abhor the idea of not being close enough to hold your baby, not for hours . . . You think about that warm, soft little body crying for *you*, and you start taking off your coat. Well, button it up again and *go*. He'll be all right—providing, of course, the baby-sitter is trustworthy.

And on this first occasion I would recommend someone you feel *emotionally* you can trust, not just someone 'who's bound to be all right because she's taken First Aid and everything . . .' So, ideally, your own mother, or a neighbour who has three children of her own and has already helped you change nappies and things for this baby.

So you see the film, overcome the urge to phone home every half-hour to make sure all is well, and yet when you do get back the sitter reports the baby was fretful, cried for his feed earlier than you said he could have it, and you feel guilty about having left him. Don't be; this is normal. What babies don't understand intellectually, they are able to sense (as we've said before) and this is the first big break with Mother. She wasn't even in the house, her presence was nowhere to be felt. But his concern is not a reason for then saying: 'Oh my poor baby missed me too much and I'll sit here until he is an adult.' No, you comfort him (if he is still protesting), and a week or so later you repeat the process until you can go out for an afternoon, even a whole day.

If your baby refuses to allow you longer than an hour (he doesn't just fret, he positively screams), or you as a mother find the very idea of leaving your child in someone else's hands too painful to contemplate, I advise you try this. Invite someone who is good with children for tea, and deliberately go away into the kitchen to get it, leaving this person in the living-room to entertain your child. Now, this recipe is of no value if your baby is fast asleep, because then this other person doesn't

E

have the opportunity of forming a relationship with him. So
choose a time when he is awake—perhaps just before or
just after a feed. It's good for him to get to know other people.
It's the first stage in being able to face those examiners without you, and it is also good for you.

A possessive mother makes for an unhappy child, and possessive mothers start out genuinely believing they are indis-
pensable to their babies, and then proceed to make this true
by jealously preventing anyone else from getting close to them
. . . including, in extreme cases, Father. 'My child,' they say, as
if their husband didn't have anything to do with it.

So if you find yourself thinking that nobody else quite knows
how to treat your baby, call for a sitter—quick.

Incidentally, it is almost as bad if your baby is tied emotionally to only one other person besides yourself, say Grandmother. Ideally he should have a small circle of friends—
whether they are blood relations or not, whom he will stay with
happily, whose attentions he will permit without fuss. And
those friends of his need not necessarily be close friends of
yours. The seventeen-year-old daughter of the family who lives
opposite may be ill-at-ease with you (perhaps because you
belong to a passé generation) but she could turn out to be
wonderful with him. Your husband's Aunt Ada may come
into her own at last. Her attitude towards babies may not be
yours. She may coo 'baby talk'; she may dotingly nurse him for
as long as he wants; she may fasten nappies differently. So
long as your baby likes her and she is a responsible person, it
doesn't matter. He'll welcome the change of pace and the rare
indulgence.

I say 'rare' because I am assuming you will be utilising
Aunt Ada or the girl opposite for comparatively short sessions.
If you're thinking in terms of a holiday, someone whose
routine and attitude are similar to yours would be infinitely
preferable, and someone from his circle whom he knows very
well indeed.

Because I am so firmly convinced of the importance of maintaining and strengthening, not only the parent-child relationship but also the husband-wife relationship, I'm all for short
holidays away from your young baby. But short is the operative

word. In general, most young mothers wouldn't enjoy a long holiday away from their babies anyway, so it's not really practical to talk about not having a three-months' holiday but a fortnight's holiday will be all right. Even a week can seem like an eternity to an eight-month-old. However good and kind and loving the person is who takes care of your baby, she is not you. Consider what it's like to a human being who cannot express his need to be with you in words, not to see you day after day; as far as he is concerned it might as well be for ever. Time is a meaningless concept at this age. He has no idea what future is and only a very sketchy memory of past. Present is everything, and at present you are absent.

So at this stage it would probably be a question of a weekend away. By the time he is a year, you could safely lengthen this to a week. But I think it should be said that during any period when a child is going to be left with another person for longer than a day, it is desirable that he become reacquainted with this person for at least a day beforehand. It also helps if the baby-sitter comes to your house, rather than Baby going to hers. This way at least his room, his cot, the wallpaper, the routine, remains the same and only the person who looks after him is different. This method may also help the baby who needs to be weaned away from you more gently than you expected—the one who yells every time his pram is parked in a strange garden. Take it one step at a time : first a friend to talk to while you're out of the room, later a baby-sitter in his house, and finally graduating to a 'day out'.

If you've been gasping to say that you don't have an Aunt Ada, nor a girl across the street, and both sets of grandparents live at the opposite end of the country—in short, you don't have *anyone* to baby-sit, let alone a circle of baby-sitters, I sympathise. Let's discuss your problem.

Have you seen anybody at all in your road with young children—not necessarily of the same age as your own baby? If so, approach her and see if you can't come to a reciprocal baby-sitting arrangement. But do be sure it *is* reciprocal. There is a vast difference between keeping an eye on a baby sleeping in his pram while his mother goes shopping, and in return entertaining three rowdy youngsters to tea while their mother goes shopping herself. This is not fair; it's like asking someone to do a job worth £10.00 and offering 50p.

At night, for a family who have three children of their own, supervising an extra baby in the house obviously involves very little extra responsibility and, providing he doesn't wake, no extra work at all. But to expect the baby's parents to have one's three children lying on various spare mattresses for an evening is hardly equal return. Some other form of payment would have to be worked out in such cases. If it isn't, the system will come to a fast and bitter end.

In the case of two neighbouring houses, it is possible to baby-sit with an alarm linked up between them. (For those of you who haven't come across this particular piece of apparatus, a baby-alarm has a microphone next to the baby's cot and a speaker in the house next door: so that the neighbours can hear the baby if he cries.) It's a very convenient method because Baby sleeps undisturbed in his own cot, and the sitters don't have to split up, so that one parent looks after the baby next door and the other their own children.

But quite frankly I don't feel entirely happy about it. I would never do it if there was a fire left on or, to a lesser degree, an electric light: because wiring behind the wainscoting has caught fire before now. You can't smell smoke and you can't see sparks through a baby-alarm; you can only hear. Under certain circumstances the baby-alarm method is workable, but for preference a sitter (Human variety) every time.

A free, reliable way of getting baby-sitters is to join a baby-sitting circle. If you live on a new housing estate, for instance, where there are a lot of young families, there is probably one in existence already. If there isn't, be the pioneer. Start one. A good person to contact is your health visitor because she will know addresses of other mothers with babies and small children who live close to you. Then get busy with an availablity list and a points system—usually one point an hour and two points for sitters after midnight. The trouble with Circles is that in order to be fair, they tend towards the bureaucratic. I've known many parents drop out because they couldn't stand the fiddling about with half-points for the odd twenty minutes. So try to be patient and see all the official recording as a necessary evil : it does prevent someone swanning home from what should have been a trip to the pictures, at 2 a.m., with the bland explanation 'they went on somewhere' !

Finally I'd like to say a word about the 'professional' baby-sitter—the person who advertises on a card outside the news-agent or in the local paper that she augments her income by baby-sitting at people's houses. Very often these sitters are elderly women, who enjoy getting out of their homes and knit-ting by your fireside or watching your television for a change, or teenagers who need some peace to study. But make no mis-take : both groups do it for money.

So first of all, find out what the standard rate for the job is. At the current moment it is somewhere between 25p and 42½p, depending on the local supply-and-demand of sitters, whether it's a weekend, how much work is involved (more if the children need a meal cooked for them, rather than if they are in bed asleep), and again whether the sitter is required after mid-night. You should expect to give the baby-sitter, in addition to her fee, some sort of supper. I don't mean she must be left the most expensive smoked salmon or steak, but it must be adequate food with enough milk, etc., for several cups of tea or coffee during her shift !

My own two daughters have both done a fair amount of professional baby-sitting, so I am quite a proxy expert on what one should and shouldn't do to the sitter. That's how I knew about the milk. My younger daughter once took care of a baby and discovered there was only about a quarter of a pint of milk in the house, and she could only find one nappy—and that after much searching. So please ensure that your baby-sitter is shown clearly where all the things are which she might need both for the baby's comfort (gripe-water, tal-cum-powder, Dentinox, nappy-bucket) and her own.

My daughters have often complained that they have sat for the whole evening wearing a coat and still shivering be-cause the small electric or gas fire was hopelessly inadequate. I have known one instance where the parents went one further : they actually requested my daughter not to sit with the light on unless she was actually reading, in order to keep the elec-tricity bill down ! If you choose to economise on your fuel in your own house, well that's your affair. But you cannot expect someone else who is employed to do a job to be uncomfortable while doing it.

It's almost expected these days that you should have a television! Do remember to show your baby-sitter how to find her way from ITV to B.B.C. and back. A quick way to spoil a beautiful sitter/parent relationship is to have the sitter miss a favourite programme because she doesn't know how the dratted TV adjusts! This applies to all things that switch on and off which she might need to use—fires, electric kettles, light-switches for the kitchen, the toilet, the landing. Allow yourselves an extra ten minutes to say all these things, because you shouldn't leave someone to grope around in half-darkness desperately searching.

And while you're about it, be sure to inform her of the household rules—one story only before sleep, or Teddy in bed and not the whole farmyard. And equally be sure the child knows them. It is not fair to leave a baby-sitter with children who are barely controllable by their own parents, because it is always that much more difficult for a stranger to impose discipline.

It is also expected that after 11 o'clock at night some form of transport will be laid on to take your baby-sitter home; you don't simply return at midnight and say to your baby-sitter, 'Well, here's your pound . . . thank you very much . . . goodnight,' and let your sitter walk back.

While saying all this, I've perhaps implied that baby-sitters are hard done by. On the whole, of course, they're not. They have a very cushy time. The child sleeps the entire time, and they have a free meal and a pound or so for doing absolutely nothing.

But do bear in mind that, like the skilled pilot of a jet plane which flies on 'George' much of the journey, you are paying them for coping with the rare emergency. So be certain that if one arises, they can handle it.

Try and meet your baby-sitter before the big day and make up your own mind that she's capable and trustworthy and that the baby will be happy with her. If she turns out to be a deaf old lady who is wobbly going up the stairs and who would be physically incapable of lifting him up, have the courage to apologise and tell her she's not really what you're looking for. After all, WE COULD BE TALKING ABOUT YOUR CHILD'S LIFE. The same applies to a fifteen-year-old who doesn't know what a bottle or a nappy look like and is only interested in a warm room where she can do a spot of necking with her boy friend. Say no.

Obviously all 'the codes of good behaviour by parents' refer just as much to the unpaid sitter (the relation or friend or member of the Circle). And so does this thing of knowing when *not* to trust. I have some amusing, sophisticated friends whose company I enjoy very much whom I wouldn't trust for five minutes in charge of a young child. I don't mean they'd pop marbles in his mouth. They wouldn't be stupid, but perhaps absent-minded. They wouldn't notice that the child they were supposed to be keeping an eye on had crawled out into the hall and was currently mounting the stairs. Don't be ashamed to admit to yourself that some of *your* friends cannot be counted as 'Friends of Baby'.

So far I have dealt with situations when *you* have to leave *your baby*. Sadly, a few babies have to leave their parents to go into hospital. Because there is more you can do to prepare him for the experience and because it is then more common, I am going to deal with this problem in the next age-group. But I would remind you that even one-year-olds understand far more than they can ever say; so talking comfortably about some key words like 'nurse' may help, and an extra dose of love beforehand may sustain him. A withdrawal of love, on the grounds that he's going to be without you for a fortnight, certainly won't.

Although we hope your baby isn't going to find out about hospital, by the time he passes out of this age-group he's an old hand with clinics, doctors, vaccination and inoculations. Nurses, often because they are busy or because they haven't considered it, will take your baby away into the surgery to give him his injection leaving you in the waiting room. Your child won't like the momentary pain of the needle whatever you do; but if you are firm and insist that you will hold him while he is having his very necessary discomfort administered, although the physical pain will be no less, the emotional pain will be much less. You see, if you stay there (and it's an important thing to keep in mind) at least you haven't abandoned him to suffer pain; you remained with him while it hurt. It's only a moment but it is perhaps one of the earliest occasions when relationship under stress will be put to the test, and it's good for a baby to know he has a mother for better and for worse.

15 months – 3 years

Let's start off on this question of a parting when your toddler has to go into hospital. First of all make sure that a parting *is* inevitable. As we've just said in the previous age-group, a child needs his mother even more when he's in pain or ill or frightened—and yet he is forced to cope without her. Fortunately, some enlightened hospitals have realised this and have started to provide facilities for mothers to rest and sleep there with their children. Mother's comfort at such a time is immeasurable; and so if your child is taken into a hospital which encourages this—providing the rest of your family can manage without you for a few days, even one day—do take advantage of the scheme.

Regrettably not all hospitals can allow this yet; but thank heaven the vast majority do now permit visiting of sick children. Once upon a time it was felt that parents upset their children because, when visiting-hour was over and they had to leave, the children screamed and protested; whilst if they never saw their parents at all, they were quiet and well-behaved —that is, seemingly calm and acquiescent. Nothing could be further from the truth. Yes, on the surface perhaps; but what the child suffered secretly by not seeing his parents for perhaps a week, a fortnight, and I have known cases for three months, cannot be assessed. There just isn't a scale by which to measure such emotional damage.

Of course it hurts to wave goodbye to someone you love; even adults cry, so no wonder small children do. But it hurts far far more to have to assume that this loved one has forgotten your very existence, doesn't it? So see your child as often as you possibly can, and on days when you personally cannot get to the hospital, find out if someone like Grandmother is able to

go instead. It's very lonely and humiliating sitting in your cot
with no one to talk to, when all the other children are surrounded by Mummies and Daddies. And when you *are* there,
be affectionate and friendly . . . and hold back any tears or
lumps-in-the-throat until you're outside again. A sure-fire
way to distress your child is by showing your own distress.

And if you are informed that in this particular hospital
children are managed more easily if they are not constantly
being disturbed by visits from home, lobby the Matron or
Hospital Management Committee fast. Tell them that children
under five may well be 'managed' more easily if parents don't
visit them, but you're not risking the ghastly consequences!

Before we leave the subject of partings due to hospitalisa-
tion, I'd like to mention the converse—when *you* have to go
into hospital. In Maternity Wards I noticed early on that 'first
mothers' were usually only too glad to have the full ten days
lying-in while experts took charge of their new arrivals; whereas women who had children already were itching for home
inside twenty-four hours. They always said they were missing
their three-year-old or their twins. Their husbands they still
saw, albeit briefly, every evening. For sound infection and
discipline reasons most hospitals forbid junior visitors; but this
is very tough on both mother and child. I remember one husband telling his wife (rather foolishly) that their four-year-old
had stormed that he hated Mummy and never wanted to see
her again. What he meant was the complete parting had been
too long for him to cope with. This is another instance when a
'lobby' to allow 'walking cases' to talk to their children on a
terrace or somewhere would do wonders.

I'd like to return now to happier reasons for being parted.
Holidays, for instance. By the time your child is eighteen
months I hope that, if you should want to, he will let you go
away for a week and, at a year older than that say, a fortnight.
But I'm afraid it's quite possible that he may be of a highly
nervous temperament, and despite your having religiously
followed my instructions, refuse to allow you out of his sight
for a single afternoon.

If the baby-sitter does report that he screamed the entire
time you were gone, always make sure first that he didn't cry

for any other reason—because of indigestion, because he had a cold coming, because he was cutting a tooth . . . Then if you're still certain, you'll have to go back to the gradient scale and work it from half an hour upwards. Create brief partings when it's not imperative, like quite deliberately leaving him with someone while you do the weekend shopping, even though you could obviously take him in the pram, to hasten his readiness to accept a separation when it is imperative.

But during this testing period, do take care that the person who stays with him is not only familiar, kind and very patient, but is also confident about having him. If he senses that *she* has doubts about whether he'll be all right in her charge, his own fears will quickly surface. The same applies to your own attitude when you return. Greet him happily and calmly . . . even if he's screaming blue murder at the time. Comfort him, of course; but be firm about it. The point to get across to him is that he's got his mummy back again and nothing irrevocably dreadful has happened to him in the meantime. Believe me, in time he will start to trust you not to abandon him for ever, and in turn he'll find out that other people's company can even have its advantages.

Incidentally, whenever you hand your child over to someone else, try not to dash off instantly. It is a bit bewildering to be dumped in the middle of a strange carpet and watch Mummy flying out of the door, shouting instructions at this new lady over her shoulder! If you can delay that changeover for five minutes or so, your child will have had time to recall that the lady is Aunt Meg and that even if the carpet's strange, they're his own bricks and trolley sitting in the middle of it.

But don't assume from that I'm advocating you should wait until he's involved with his bricks and then sneak off. I am strongly against backing out quietly. It is anti-social (and therefore setting a bad example) and it also causes alarm when he does look up and miss you some twenty minutes afterwards. If you are weaning him away from total dependence on you sufficiently gradually, you should never meet a situation where you have to retreat out the back door while a small somebody is loudly banging and drumming the front one! So: say good-bye, tell him you're going to buy a pretty new dress and you'll see him at teatime. And if he barely glances up in response, bully for you. You can think about that week's holiday.

If you do go away without your toddler—unlike the baby who prefers the routine and surroundings he knows—you may find that this older child would welcome a change: a bit of a holiday of his own. He might like the 'difference' of living by the sea with Grandmother or in the country with Aunt Meg. But the object of *his* going *there* is convenience for the sitter and pleasure for him, not 'to get him away from anything that might remind him of Mummy and Daddy'. There is no reason to suppose that forgetting he has parents will benefit any child. Quite the reverse: the lesson to be learnt is that he does have a mother and a father and that they can still love one another even though they're not together.

It may sound callous, but in my opinion it is even worth having a small scene by refreshing his memory about Mummy and Daddy, because it is simultaneously reassuring that they are around somewhere and care about him.

For this reason I'd send him a couple of postcards. He'll look at the pictures, but don't expect your message to have the same value that it would to an eight-year-old. Even when it is explained to him that 'This is from Mummy and Daddy, and they send you lots and lots of love and kisses, and they'll be back soon,' the child cannot understand intellectually what this means. Yet he can understand emotionally. He will hear the cheerfulness in Grandma's voice as she mentions Mummy and Daddy and, on a non-verbal level, he will be reassured that all is well.

If you have difficulty in grasping this, remember back to when you were in the flush of your first love and how you used to sit quietly and repeat his name over and over again to yourself. 'John . . . John . . . John . . .' Just saying the name or hearing somebody else mention a John, not even your John, gave you an emotional feeling of warmth and love, because the sound evoked certain associations. Well, now the same thing applies to a young child. There is an ambience of security, love and happiness to him about the words 'Mummy' and 'Daddy'.

So far I have discussed only baby-sitting on an irregular basis, mainly for social reasons. Now I'd like to talk about baby-minding or child-minding as a daily routine while Mother goes out to work.

I omitted the working mother from the previous age-group because, as you will have gathered, I believe a child should not be asked to accept long partings from Mother during his first year. I have kept stressing that word 'gradual', and it is not gentle weaning to be placed with a baby-minder for five hours from Monday to Friday. If you have to work for pressing economic reasons—and by pressing I mean you honestly can't meet the food bill by Wednesday—that's different. Like the child who seldom sees his father owing to his business-hours, it's sad but it has to be endured.

No, I'm speaking of the wife who yearns for the career life too, or who desires the extras, like a spin-drier or a proper holiday, that the income from a part-time job may provide.

It is not the purpose of this book either to advocate or oppose the working mother. Whether or not a woman wants to go to work is something she has to figure out for herself, if necessary with the aid of her husband. It is, however, true to say that there is nothing worse than a mother who feels frustrated at being cooped up at home with small children and is so busy dreaming of the 'greener grass' she doesn't enjoy the time she spends with her young family. Consciously or subconsciously, she may very well come to blame them for her 'imprisonment' and that makes for an unhappy mother/child relationship. If she tells them of her resentment, she'll distress them; if she keeps it to herself, she'll turn into a martyr. Thus it is better for this woman to go out to work and use the money she earns paying for child-care.

I was one of these myself. With each of my three children, I recognised that as they emerged from babyhood we weren't really having fun together. I wasn't appreciating being a mother because I was constantly aware of the lack of adult company, of stimulation. So I compromised. When my first baby was around a year old, I took a part-time job. I used an official baby-minder for four hours a day. I didn't get any financial benefit from it because most of what I earned went on my lunches, my fares and what I had to pay the baby-minder. But I welcomed the break from being a housewife and, funnily enough, began to look forward to getting back home again. All in all I enjoyed my toddler much more, and I'm sure she enjoyed me, now I was no longer irritated by her existence.

Let me say quickly that there is no implication that the woman who is quite content to be at home looking after her children, the woman who would rather suffer some economic hardship than leave them regularly in someone else's care, is not just as good a mother and person. She is. I have a daughter who is in exactly this position. She had an interesting job before she was married but now she is completely satisfied, at the age of twenty-three, to be simply a housewife and a mother of a young baby. And an excellent job she's making of her role, too.

What I'm sure *is* undesirable is being unable to come to terms with how one feels about this career/motherhood question, and therefore either being frustrated at home or feeling violently guilty because one has, in one's own opinion, abandoned the children. So you must discuss the problem, make a decision . . . and then live with it without miserable periods of introspection and remorse.

I'm not here speaking of extremes. I'm not referring to the woman who is so possessive she cannot bear anyone to take her place even temporarily and who uses 'maternal dedication' as an excuse for ceasing to be a wife or indeed a human being. Nor do I mean the woman who goes out to work leaving her children to roam about with a latch-key round their necks and vague instructions to knock on Mrs. Jones's door if they want anything. We're thinking of the moderate, responsible woman who makes a compromise which suits both herself and her children.

It's possible that you could pair off with a mother who belongs to the opposite brigade—i.e. while you work, pay a friend who is choosing to stay at home with her own children to take care of your offspring as well. (Or vice versa.) (See 'Your Child and The Law', page 241.) But if that isn't 'on', then you'll have to utilise a professional baby-minder.

Make sure that she is registered with the Local Authority, because that ensures her care is up to a certain standard. Even so, I think I would make a point of enrolling my child during her working hours with other children, so that one can see for oneself that she is a kind, sensible person with a hygienic set-up.

Needless to say, if your child resists in any sense whenever he approaches or is left with the baby-minder, I'm afraid you will just have to resign from your job and, once again, work up to this sort of separation more gradually—if you have your child's welfare at heart, that is. As I've said : you are not a bad mother just because you want a career as well; you are, if you allow this need to damage your child psychologically.

So if your child remains playful, responsive, boisterous, greets you gladly but calmly when you come back, then all is well. But beware of the converse of any of these things, or if your child undergoes changes in temperament that you cannot justify simply by the fact he is growing up—for instance, if a normally contented extrovert child turns into an irritable introverted one. Or if he suddenly falls victim to feeding-troubles, skin-sensitivity, disturbed sleep at night or returns to pants-wetting. These physical irregularities could have emotional roots. He may be suffering from loneliness or fear you've rejected him because, where once you stayed with him you now hand him over to a baby-minder.

It is only fair to point out that if you ignore these symptoms of your toddler's insecurity, the trouble may not show immediately but instead manifest itself later, when the earlier incident is no longer obvious. As you have doubtless noticed, I like to avoid laying the foundation of trouble. I much prefer to show you how to prevent problems than to have to tell you what to do after they have arisen. In this I apparently differ from many experts in the child-care field, who are busy telling parents how to cope with *disturbed* children !

All this being so, the last thing I want to do is to alarm you into quitting your job at the first hint of a missed meal or a cross mood. Give yourselves a fair chance. Before claiming he cannot cope with the baby-minder, make absolutely certain the irritability isn't just a crotchety week (even the nicest

among us have them), or the skin-disorder merely a passing
heat-rash.

3 – 5 years

This is the period when your child will be off your hands at
playgroup and nursery school, and you may be tempted to take
on a larger part-time or even a full-time job. I would warn
you, though, that you may find a job combined with your
cleaning and shopping and washing and gardening, plus the
physical care of a four-year-old, so exhausting that when you
collect your child each afternoon all you can afford to do in
terms of energy is give him a hurried tea and dump him in his
bed. This obviously will not do. The child wouldn't have a
mother to cuddle, and play with and talk to. He'd barely see
her . . . only at breakfast as she dashed about organising her
busy day and then again for half an hour in the evening as
she shooed him off to bed. Certainly he would see you at weekends, but I've known far too many working mothers who were
so tired by Saturday all they wanted to do was sink down in
an armchair.

If you haven't the stamina for career and motherhood, I
strongly recommend you select the latter. (It's a little late for
you now to do otherwise.) There is plenty of opportunity after
the range of this book, when your child is away seven hours
daily at proper school, for pursuing a career. There is only *now*
for shaping your child's emotional background.

Even if *you* can cope with, say, a six-hour working day, it
is still very possible your child will be unable to do so. He may
have adored his daily two hours at play-group but find a full
morning at nursery school followed by an afternoon with the
child-minder too long a separation from you. He may tell you
so; but if he doesn't, how will you know?

Well, to give you an example, if he has been the bouncy,
mischievous piece of humanity we all know as a happy child
who feels secure in the love of his parents, and he suddenly
becomes quiet and hardly seems to take an interest in what's
going on around him—beware. Most particularly take warning if the child-minder reports how *good* he is, meaning he
sits obediently in a chair all afternoon. Normal children are not

like that; they want to be interested in something, active and, to a degree, 'try it on'. So the child who is sitting quietly is actually withdrawing into himself, probably because he is deeply distressed.

Equally if your child plays all day, laughs, eats, but as soon as you appear he becomes angry, fretful, even violent—again, look out. Don't assume he loves nursery school so much he doesn't want to leave it. If that was so, he'd complain but still be glad to see you. No, in fact he is punishing you for having left him ... *deserted* him.

I can only say in general terms: observe your child, and listen to the experienced advice of his play-group leader or nursery-school teacher. If you and they are confident that he is happy, then nothing could be better for him than the child-orientated environment of Playgroup or nursery school. It stimulates him; it gives him friends; it prepares him for the essential coming break of proper school. Whether or not he attends a child-minder's too will, of course, depend on the decision you reached—you know, the decision you were going to live with without introspection and remorse.

Of course, since the war more and more families have been taking on a 'living-in child-minder': an *au pair* girl.

If you have never had an *au pair* living in your home or never had close experience of a household where one was employed, I think you should be warned about certain aspects of this seemingly attractive solution. First of all the *au pair* doesn't come principally because she's interested in helping you take care of your children. She comes because she wants to travel and learn English, and this is a cheap way of doing it. She may, if you're lucky, do her work satisfactorily in order to carry out the conditions of her contract; but that's all. The job was never meant to be her chosen career. At best, she'll teach your children to speak English with a Swedish accent. At worst, I fear that after the novelty of being in a different country and a new home has worn off, after she has found a boy friend and a social life of her own, she will become indifferent.

There are exceptions. I readily admit that there are some superb girls—often daughters of large families themselves, who genuinely love children and prove to be gifts from heaven. But these are rare. And don't forget you usually take an *au pair* 'sight unseen' from the boat; so you don't have an opportunity of picking the angel from a bunch of very mortal girls!

And is a young foreigner the most reliable person to leave in charge of young children anyway? Certainly she can sit in a living-room and watch for fires while they are asleep upstairs; she can know when it's 10 o'clock and time to give the baby his bottle. But can she cope all day long on her own, or with a crisis in the middle of the night? Bear in mind she's a stranger in a strange country, and that country has unfamiliar customs and an unfamiliar language.

There can also be emotional complications with an *au pair* girl. There are so many jokes about husbands going off with the French *au pair*, you can't have failed to have thought of that one! But just consider the strain caused by the intrusion of a third party on a faithful, happy marriage. Remember, she is a *guest*, not a servant who can be banished to her room whenever you and your husband want to be alone. She will be there when she wants to be there, and that's whenever she hasn't anything more exciting to do outside. She'll be sitting with you both for your evening meal—probably the first chance you and your husband have had to talk to each other that day—and she'll be around for the rest of the evening when you want to relax in front of the television. It can get awfully tiresome.

Finally, *au pairs* are a transitory breed. Unless yours is very exceptional, she won't stay with you for very long. And nothing is harder on your child than to have an *au pair* with whom, because she is young and superficially friendly, he starts an affectionate relationship only to find three months later she has left him and he is expected to adjust to a completely new girl. And this process is repeated over and over and over again. We've said before: children need continuity in their relationships, and an *au pair* can seldom supply this.

There is, however, a permanent alternative to an *au pair*, and that is to employ a professional nanny. I am well aware that such a suggestion is outside the economic possibilities of most of us. Nannies are highly trained for their work and demand a relative high salary, not to mention their own room,

etc. But there are among my readers, people who, because
their jobs are so important to them, or because they genuinely
feel so incapable of, or so unfitted for, the role of housewife
and mother, would prefer to plough back their own earnings into paying someone skilled to take over their domestic
role.

It sometimes works very well, too. Nannies are usually
people who love children, which is why they chose this career.
In purely practical terms also, they have much more know-
how than the average mother, who learns by trial and error
on the poor eldest of her children. Nanny learns all about
nappy-changing and table-manners before she comes. Incidentally, this very fact has its disadvantages. She has her own
way of doing things, often rather strict ways, and you would
have to accept them. That has to be the understanding : Nanny
is in sole charge from Monday to Friday (perhaps with
Mother returning home from her job in time to kiss
the children goodnight) and the parents take over at weekends.

I've noticed that very often these parents try to compensate
for their lengthy absence by being extra special 'fun' parents
when they are there. Saturdays and Sundays are absolutely
packed with treats—tea-parties, visits to the zoo, outings to the
sea, family games, all accompanied by the sort of luxury
presents ordinary children receive only once or twice a year. I'm
not quarrelling with the belief that this arrangement thrills the
children and allows the parents to give them unstinting attention for two whole days. Trouble is, you know : they demote
themselves to Favourite Aunt and Uncle.

The sort of attachment most children form for Mother
has had to be given to Nanny. She's the one who's always
there; she's the person the child automatically goes to for
his daily needs—because he is hurt, because he's unhappy,
because he has a pain, because he is hungry; he can't sleep;
he wants to sleep . . . So if you're contemplating a professional
nanny face up to the penalty now. You mustn't feel jealous
or wounded if, when your child cries, he cries for Nanny.

To sum up, let me say this. Although through history all the
people we know about (the people from the aristocracy whose

names have been handed down to us as great people) were all nanny-reared, I firmly believe the ideal is still a home with a loving, amateur mother and father in it and not a nanny-dominated nursery however well-organised it might be.

CHAPTER EIGHT

Who's Afraid of the Big Bad Wolf?

I suppose we'd all be afraid if confronted by a snarling pack of wolves in the middle of a lonely forest. That sort of fear is logical, essential even to our survivial. But constantly to fear the possibility of encountering a wild wolf when one lives in the heart of an English city, that's *il*logical. We call that sort of fear a phobia. Young children are particular victims of phobias, and so I want to devote a whole chapter to the subject.

The first thing to say about phobias is that, although they're nonsense to the outsider, to the sufferer they are only too real. The main thing to remember in every case of phobia attack is that the immediate circumstance is the trigger of the phobia, and the phobia itself, whatever it may consist of, is based upon fear of an unknown quantity.

If you yourself fear spiders or snakes or waterfalls, you will know what I'm talking about. You will understand that it only makes it worse if you are told not to be stupid and made to fight it out. Equally, if you're over-protected from meeting the experience you dread, you'll never have a chance to get used to it and conquer it.

Personally I am terrified of thunderstorms. Now, if someone had stood me out in the middle of a field or, at that, forced me to stand by a picture-window while a thunderstorm was in progress, I would probably be even more frightened of them than I am. As you gather, no one did.

Instead my mother went to the other extreme. She, too, was terrified of thunderstorms and whenever one started, she would crawl under the dining-room table with a blanket over her head and me clasped to her bosom. Small wonder I still have this phobia. I did have enough restraint, though, not to continue this dubious practice as far as my own children were concerned and, sure enough, they are not nervous about thunderstorms. They know about not tempting disaster by standing under a solitary tree, but they certainly have no illogical fear of thunder and lightning. In fact they happily count the interval between flash and roar and discuss the scientific possibilities. I, meanwhile, stay with the cat and the dog, because it is generally agreed in our household that it's best for the scared ones to keep together!

Incidentally, in the course of controlling myself and my behaviour during storms while my children were small and impressionable, I have overcome a good deal of my own fear.

It's important, I think, to say here that you're not a failure as a parent just because your child is aware you have a phobia. It's only if you infect him with it that it's bad. It may even be a good thing for him to learn early on that you're only human, and that he must be considerate of your fears just as you're considerate of his. This is up to Father. He must explain that Mummy is afraid of (in my case, mice) and that we therefore never tease her with them. (Cancel that advice if Father is a sadistic practical joker!)

I never minded the children knowing I was frightened of house-mice—after all, now you know it, too. But I couldn't rationalise for them *why* I was frightened. I still can't. I have handled white laboratory mice without repulsion; I stroke 'bigger mice' like guinea pigs; but show me a brown mouse which has bored a hole in the larder and I can only just stop the scream. I've found that observing one from a safe distance, with the knowledge I can always retreat, and the next day coming a little closer to it does help me to come to terms with my phobia.

And this, I firmly believe, is the method one should adopt in teaching one's children to overcome *their* strange fears. Always use a gradual approach. He may fear the budgerigar or a new house or a hanging lamp with a curious fringed crimson shade. Let him examine it at a distance before he comes close, and the moment you see more signs of 'Ah, ah: I don't know what this is—help!', stop, retreat a step, comfort and reassure. Then the next day try again.

It is generally true to say that if you yourself are of an anxious temperament, if you tend to worry about things which most of your friends would take in their stride, this anxiety does pervade the atmosphere and will tend to produce an anxious child. Well, at least you'll be sympathetic to his fears, which does to some extent compensate him for not being the robust, daring little fellow your friends have produced.

Sometimes, of course, the Fates are really unkind and issue those outgoing, happy-go-lucky parents who welcome challenges with a child who is the exact opposite. If you are in this situation, I beg you to show extra understanding to your sensitive, withdrawn little'un. He has his contribution to make as a human being, but if you try to force him to make it your way, bravely and heartily, you could very easily break him completely.

So let's now talk in detail about some of the more common phobias of early childhood and how to deal with them. Obviously there will be many, many others for which I haven't room in this book. On those I'd give the old advice : watch your own child and apply the gradient scale.

0 – 3 months

A baby under three months may be frightened of a weird-looking mobile hanging over his cot or a bizarre wallpaper on his nursery wall. If he screams, pick him up soothingly and carry him away from whatever upset him. But the best way to combat this sort of phobia is to avoid it. If a trendy young aunt buys him a grotesque gonk as a birth gift, put it away in a cupboard until your child is old enough to think it funny. And don't choose a room for your nursery that has a loud paper that might scare him. Remember that if he's born in hospital, he may well spend the first ten days of his life looking at plain cream walls. Quite a shock, therefore, coming home to scarlet and purple whirls !

Another one with young babies is a sudden loud noise, like a door banging or the very shrill ring of a telephone. Obviously you cannot live in a tomb and if your door is given to banging and the other members of the family tend to forget this, then your poor baby is going to be exposed to his phobia over and over again. You can try a notice on the door saying : 'PLEASE CLOSE GENTLY', but if I know families they won't even see it after the first week! You'd do better to move Baby's cot away from the front door or the phone and organise it so that he is sleeping, whether in the daytime or in the evening, as far from the source of the noise as possible.

And when he does cry in terror, comfort him *calmly*. Gradually he'll get the message that no one else around is frightened, and so perhaps there's nothing to be frightened of. And in any case, as a child grows older his nervous system becomes accustomed to noise, even sudden noise; so in this instance he really will grow out of it.

3 – 9 months

Unfortunately while he outgrows those fears, he acquires others. He may become frightened of new people, or young men, or men in uniform, coloured people if he is unused to coloured people (incidentally, I'm told that some coloured children who never or rarely see white people have the same reaction to a pink face), people with white hair, a person wearing glasses—especially dark glasses or glasses with heavy frames.

Now if, for instance, when Granny wears her heavy-framed glasses, the child stiffens and screams with fear, there is no point in Granny continuing to hold him clasped tightly to her breast. That's like the lion holding you in his teeth to reassure you he's not going to bite. You have that nagging doubt that at any moment he could change his mind! You'd kind of rather he put you down and then told you. Same with Granny. The thing to do is for the child to be removed and for Granny to take off the glasses. Then the child can observe her from a distance and approach when he feels ready.

Many a baby under the age of a year is frightened if a human face comes too close, it's enormous to him. Yes, even if the face is making cooing noises and smiling. That's why we, as parents, have to try to keep our loving friends and relatives at a slight distance from the baby, particularly if he has just woken up, particularly if he doesn't know them, and particularly if they're wearing something which he might take exception to, like a large hat.

It's possible, too, that he can suddenly be scared stiff of you. A young mother told me that one day she picked up her baby and he stiffened (that's usually the clue symptom to this sort of fear), screamed and tried to get away from her. 'It's Mummy,' she kept saying, cuddling him, and the more she cuddled him, the more frantic he became. Eventually she gave up trying to soothe him and put him in his high-chair for his tea. (Unconsciously removing him a few inches from his *bête noire*.) He was now able to be sufficiently reassured by her familiar voice and the routine of eating to stop crying; nevertheless he kept a wary eye on something just above her head. She examined the wall behind her, the ceiling, and suddenly realised what it was: she was wearing hair-rollers, and he had never seen Mummy looking like a geisha girl or a Martian. She did the only sensible thing one can do in the circumstances. She took out one of the yellow plastic rollers to prove that it was harmless. She played with it, showing him it was light and could roll about, and finally he dared to hold it. But he took all that convincing that Mummy was really Mummy, and even if she was that she didn't have a monster side to her.

Another little thing that often frightens babies is if a piece of furniture is not in its accustomed place in the room, or if their cot has been moved so that they see the room from an unexpected angle. So if you find your baby suddenly goes rigid and screams for no apparent physical or emotional reason, look around. What have you done? What have you moved? What has changed? What is there that wasn't there before?

The play of light and shadow on a cupboard against the window can seem like a menacingly black shape to him. A carelessly-dropped coat on the edge of an armchair can look like a person, and a grotesque person at that. A large coloured garden umbrella can cut him off from the world he recognises. *You* know what a sun brolly is; you probably bought it so that your baby could lie outside in his carry-cot and still be comfortably shaded from the sun. But to him, unless he is carefully introduced to it, it can seem to be a threat. So if he resists, don't leave him to its mercy, strapped down with this mushroom looming above him. Let him examine it with you, and every time he refuses to look at it, take him away and let him look at it from a distance. It may take a few days; and you may fail even then. You may have to get rid of the umbrella; you may have to move the cupboard back into its original position; you may have to stop the family slinging their coats around. But it's worth giving in to keep your baby happy. Never dismiss his phobia as silly, and say he will just have to get over it. That's downright cruel, and it probably won't succeed anyway.

Just now I mentioned that he likes his cot where he expects his cot to be. You'll sympathise if you've ever woken to find yourself facing a wall when your bed at home is beside a low window. For a second there's a panic 'Where am I?' until you remember you're staying with friends. But suppose you weren't an adult who could work that out . . . Then the panic would linger, wouldn't it? Solution: don't move the nursery furniture about 'for a change' the way you do in the lounge.

It's not only the view either. He likes the familiarity of the cot itself. (Babies and infants are unashamedly conservative about most things!) So when the time comes to transfer him into the big cot, stand the cradle or carry-cot or whatever in the dropside cot at nights for a week; that way he'll grow used to his new environment. He'll regard the dropside cot as a bed and not as some vast cage with blankets.

The same applies to the promotion to the big bath. To start with, make the change-over by putting his baby bath in the big one. Or you can utilise the sink as an intermediary stage—from baby bath to kitchen sink to big bath, because that is also a gradient.

Now, just as babies are initially afraid of being bathed in a shiny white, or coloured, tank, they also often distrust their first glimpse of the seaside. A baby who is perfectly happy crawling all over the kitchen floor and the sitting-room carpet, even the lawn, may sit petrified on a beautiful sandy beach. Well, think of the noise of the sea and not understanding what it is, and this vast expanse of dun-coloured floor which is of a different substance from the lino and wool and grass he's used to. They're solid; this isn't.

So before he starts wailing inconsolably, I recommend you spread down a blanket—a small blanket which he knows, perhaps his own baby blanket—and indicate to him that this is his territory. He will feel safe on the blanket and he can examine beyond his frontiers in his own time.

9 months – 2 years

Some toddlers, too, are none too happy beside the sea. Again, it's too vast for them. I'm sure you've seen an eighteen-month-old standing alone in the middle of the sand, his mouth puckered, his eyes searching desperately for a face he knows. So to start with, he also may need to remain within the confines of your 'camp'—the circle of deckchairs, buckets, lilo, clothes, etc., and venture out only when he can hold your hand.

I have already touched upon the under fives' common phobia about moving water, when we discussed swimming in our chapter on physical development. I would add to this that if you don't live at the coast, the mere sight of swirling sea would be a totally new experience for your child; so take it gently. Personally I would first introduce him to the local paddling pool in the park, then work up to the children's end of the municipal swimming-pool, and eventually progress to the sea. And need I repeat : at any sign of fear—crying, clutching you or, more serious, going stiff and silent—you come out of the water and try again a few days later.

I also mentioned in passing, this time in connection with discipline, the child who becomes afraid of the dark. Just because your toddler used to sleep perfectly happily without a light on doesn't mean he's kidding you now. As his environment and knowledge increase, so regrettably do the number of things he's afraid of. The old argument that everybody sleeps in the dark one day and so the child had better stop this nonsense now, and with this the parent closes the door on him, is unkind and unnecessary. You won't cure him like that, and in fact *you* don't need to cure him at all. He will cure himself providing he isn't abandoned to his fear at this tender age.

A nightlight, a soft *electric* nightlight which gives a glow to his room but is not bright enough to be disturbing, or simply a landing or hall light left on is usually enough. It may even be sufficient to have the bedroom door ajar so that he has the background comfort of hearing voices, water running, the television. It will let him know there are people out there— people who will protect him from this black abyss.

2 – 5 years

I have talked a lot about agoraphobia—fear of open spaces: the baby who feels insecure in too large a cot, the toddler who doesn't like being alone on a huge beach. This age-group also suffer from it. Many small children feel completely comfortable only in a small enclosed space. That's why the Wendy House is so popular. Its appeal is partly playing house, of course, but I think it's just as much because the room is a size they can handle. As a caravaner of long experience I can state how often we had small visitors from neighbouring caravans purely because my two younger children slept in a little tent. All the children loved crawling into this warm enclosure and, once inside, they would curl up on the sleeping bags and you could practically see them expanding they were so relaxed.

But for some children this desire for small spaces is an obsession. A friend of mine who has a lot to do with nursery education told me that she once had a little girl who was a chronic agoraphobiac. They had a number of wooden boxes in the nursery which were used for various games and for tables at milk-time. Well, this pupil couldn't face the threatening situation of making social contact with people other than her parents—not continually, anyway, and so she'd retreat into one of the boxes. It must have been dark and cramped for her, but there she sat for long periods. Then she would suddenly come out, play for a short while and be quite happy, and then she'd climb back into her box again.

Now, it would have been very tempting to insist that, since she enjoyed being with the other children, she stay out and involve herself in the group activity. But my friend, who knows a thing or two about children, understood that the little girl herself would decide when she no longer required what friend Freud would call 'the womb symbol'. She very wisely left her to it, and I'm glad to report that over the months the child needed her box less and less. She now seems to be very well integrated into the class; she's laughing and splashing and is just as active and makes just as much noise as the other children. So if your child develops a habit of playing in a dim corner, don't fish him out; don't even coax him out. Just be welcoming when he does emerge, and keep a casual eye on him over the next year to make sure he is returning to his corner less and less frequently rather than more and more. If the latter is true, then there is something radically wrong in his world, and you both need expert help.

I don't want to seem depressing, but for every infant *agoraphobiac*, there are probably two *claustrophobiacs*—children who fear confined spaces. Perhaps a baby-sitter has gone to the cupboard under the stairs to get out the vacuum-cleaner and the child has trotted after her. And this woman has said in fun, because many adults don't know what to say to children, 'How would it be if we pushed you back in there instead of the vacuum? Would you like to sit in there with the door closed?' They wouldn't dream of carrying this out, but the very suggestion can be enough to set off a horrible train of thought in the child's mind.

And at the risk of appalling you still further, some women even use 'locking him up' as a method of controlling a child. 'If you don't behave, I'll put you in the broom cupboard . . .' Do you wonder, incidentally, that I said choose your sitter with care!

Once a child does suffer from claustrophobia, it's very hard to cure. Many *adults* are grappling with the problem without success. That's why I'm so hot on preventing it in the first place. However, if your child, through no fault of yours, does develop this phobia, I can only suggest the obvious: promise him faithfully that you'd never leave him in the cupboard under the stairs . . . if that's what's worrying him particularly. Show him conversationally that there's a light there anyway. And bear with him about taking the escalator instead of the lift in stores and not exploring caves on holiday. With calmness and forethought on your part and a growing trust on his, he may have a fighting chance of overcoming his morbid fear.

To turn to a less drastic one. Almost all children of this age hate having their hair washed. I know *I* used to bellow like a small bull I was so scared of getting my face wet. Non-sting shampoo has quietened many of the loudest complaints but there still remains the business of water gushing over one's face and threatening to drown one. After battling with each of my own three children, I found a way round it. I placed a kitchen chair in front of the wash-basin in the bathroom and stood with one foot firmly on the chair and the child lying backwards across my thigh with his head in the basin. It's a crude imitation of the way the girl shampoos in the hairdresser's. But it works, because his face is no longer close to the water and so it's much less frightening. Admittedly you can only use one hand for washing (the other arm grasping the child round the chest to stop him slipping off), but I reckon that's easier, and certainly more pleasant, than struggling with a yelling victim.

We should, I feel, cover nightmares in this chapter. A child of two or two-and-a-half may well wake screaming from a bad dream and fail to appreciate that this nasty experience didn't happen in reality. The trouble is at that age he's unlikely to articulate clearly: he won't be able to tell you something buzzed at him and hurt him and he couldn't get away. He'll more probably just sob and, at best, mutter: 'Bee . . . bee . . .' It's up to you to catch on.

Comfort him until he's soothed but, equally important, explain about dreams in principle. Tell him that while he's in bed pictures are produced in his head and it's like watching television while he's asleep. He may see himself and Mummy in the park or the animals from his picture-book playing together; but he only pictures these things. And the funny thing about dreams is that the pictures are all jumbled up together. (By then he will understand about pictures being jumbled up because he will have played games like Snap where one can shuffle the cards and mix together all the pictures.)

He'll also be relieved to know that everybody sees pictures when they're asleep, not just him, and some of the pictures are nice and some of them are not very nice; some of them are remembered and some aren't.

As far as I know, dreams are liable to be an imponderable only with a first child, because second and subsequent children

hear older brothers and sisters talk about them. I know from
my own children that my youngest looked forward to having
a dream because it was a sort of sign of being older.

A totally different sort of phobia children have is over certain foods. They object violently to something you serve, and
it's nothing to do with the flavour; it's the *texture*. For them,
it conjures up disgusting associations. Spinach feels like slime,
macaroni like worms, etc. When this happens, I advise you
quietly to take it away from him and then exclude it from his
diet in future. Curiously enough, the association may
be subconscious; he may not have the vocabulary to express
why he hates his hard-boiled egg so much. You will recognise
it's a texture phobia only from the magnitude of the reaction,
which is a far cry from 'I don't like potatoes; they're dull.' And
unlike the potatoes that come around at the next meal regardless, hard-boiled eggs never darken his plate again. That doesn't
mean the rest of the family can't eat them. They should, because, apart from the fact they've a right to, it gives the child
an opportunity to say one day: 'Well, I suppose I could have a
little egg—not much, just a little . . .' And of course, this is the
child's instinctive way of using a gradient scale to master his
phobia.

In conclusion I would repeat something I said at the outset: that *your* anxiety fans his. This applies to physical upsets
as well as psychological. There's a golden rule for when your
child bangs his head or scrapes a knee. Wait! Wait for the
child's own reaction to his injury. If he dusts himself down,
picks himself up and carries on, swallow your concern and do
something else. If he cries because he really has hurt himself,
he really is in pain, go and give sympathetic but firm and
friendly help, and administer whatever first aid—a kiss better
or something more practical—is necessary.

I've discovered sticky-plaster is not only a protection for a
graze, but it's also almost a badge of battle. I've used many
pieces of sticky-plaster in places which weren't injured enough
to make it necessary. It works on a similar principle as the
teething-jellies, mentioned on page 75. Give it a try; it's worth
the waste of plaster.

Now, suppose you've been reading this chapter very carefully and you have grown more and more discouraged as you went along. You have a child who is a coward about his wounds; he's frightened of the dark; he's scared of strangers; he's terrified of water and confined spaces and, in addition, he has a few phobias of his very own which I haven't mentioned at all. Your husband considers the child is weak and accuses you of spoiling or pampering and, if it's a boy, perhaps he even despises him as a 'sissy'. What do you do to toughen him up, to breach this gulf between your menfolk?

You accept. You accept you have a highly-sensitive child who needs extra loving, not doubting. For whatever your husband may or may not say in the child's presence, your child will be well aware of his attitude. And to feel a failure to the parents he loves on top of being frightened of almost every new experience must be unbearable. It would drive him further into himself instead of out into that brave little daredevil your husband, and perhaps you, were hoping for. So you love him as he is, and you use the gradual reach-withdraw mechanism I've referred to throughout this chapter to cope with his many fears. And who knows?—with the spur of *your own and your husband's approval,* he may even win a few of his wars.

CHAPTER NINE

It's Getting To Be a Habit . . .

I WANT to take a brief look at those 'bad habits' children so often develop and what we, as parents, should do about them.

Comforters

The need for a comforter of some sort usually starts early. Sucking is instinctive to everyone, and no adult can say with certainty how much sucking-time as distinct from milk-taking time any one baby needs. This is where a comforter comes in. The comforter seems to be a means towards achieving a feeling of relaxation and contentment and, if nothing else is available, the baby will use his own thumb, forefinger, the tops of two fingers, or any of several combinations of these. It is known to many experts that some babies suck thumbs or forefingers while still in the womb; this is where the habit begins.

You will notice that children, and indeed many adults, sleep in a position very similar to the one they had in the womb. In other words, sleep in one respect is a retreat, a return to the safe world in which they spent so many vital months in development. But your baby can't reach this haven of safety unless he has as many factors representing the womb-like state as possible : darkness, firm wrapping, being well-fed, content, *and lying in the same position, curled and sucking finger, etc.*

The trouble with sucking thumbs or fingers is that thumbs or fingers can be (a) a source of mouth and stomach infection, (b) lead to misshapen fingers, (c) cause badly formed gums because of the hard pressure of a finger or thumb against them. So for the baby under six months which has an extra need to suck, fingers and thumbs are undesirable. *But more undesirable still is to deprive him of what he needs.*

Solution : the much-maligned *dummy.* The baby who has enough security, loving, food, is not in pain or ill, will tend to want a dummy only when he is tired or just before falling asleep. So don't imagine the horrible picture of baby lying permanently with a dummy stuck in his mouth—which is as abhorrent to me as it is to you. And if your baby needs a dummy, keep two, so that even when one is in use, there's always another being sterilised in the Milton solution with the bottle, teats and plastic spoons.

As your baby gets to be older than six months, he may prefer a 'companion/comforter'. This could be something like a muslin nappy or a dearly-loved stuffed rabbit. He hasn't got the makings of a neurotic because he refuses to settle without this companion/comforter. He'll grow up perfectly normal providing you indulge him in this—even to the extent of packing Bunny or his cloth when he spends a night away. Do not ever try to create the substitute by confiscating the cloth and replacing it with the socially far more acceptable toy. He will make the replacement when he is ready for it. Yes, even if this is not until he is four.

If your under-five seeks his comforter when he's up and about, that can be more serious. Can be. I happen to know a two-year-old who drags his muslin nappy along where other children would take their Teddy bear. This little boy is perfectly well-adjusted; he simply regards 'Bibby' (it's got some such name) as a companion. And who are we to say that a square of material hasn't got a face, a body and two arms and therefore cannot possibly be a companion ? Even so, apart from the hygiene aspect (dragging 'Bibby' through the mud and then nuzzling it is far from ideal), such dependence on any one thing is to be discouraged. Just as we, as mothers, have weaned our toddler away from our constant companionship by occasionally leaving him with a sitter, so he should, if possible, be weaned away from his rabbit's ear or muslin nappy. Try leaving it in his bed (ready for sleep-time) when he comes into the living-room to play. You may be surprised to find he'll be so engrossed with his pull-along trolley, he won't even miss it.

F

If he does and shows signs of stress, then best let him have it back. He obviously needs some sort of security prop. And that, in one sentence, is why a continual need for a comforter is serious : it means there's something in his life that makes him insecure. Find out what that is, and put it right; and the comforter will be dispensed with after a time.

In the same way thumb-sucking during the day may be a security prop. On the other hand it may just be something to do because a child is bored. One never sees a child who is happily occupied sucking his thumb. So if you have a thumb-sucker, ask yourself : are the toys he's been offered the wrong sort to stimulate *him*? (This is particularly true of a story you may be telling him : it's too difficult, or too boringly easy, and so he reckons he'll suck his thumb instead of paying attention.) Have you inadvertently made him too passive : insisting that he sit quietly with a picture-book or a box of dominoes for a large part of his day?

Of course, never smack a child for sucking his thumb. This would only make him do it secretly, and that would make the habit more obsessive than ever.

With the child who sits thumb-sucking in a corner of his cot instead of sleeping, I suspect the answer is plain : he's fed up to the back teeth—if you'll pardon the expression—with his cot. He's obviously having more rest than he needs, and instead of screaming his complaint at you, he's gone all apathetic about it. So beware. If your child continually (say, for over a week) doesn't sleep for one particular rest period, sorry, but he's cut that one out.

Now, if you're wailing that your child no longer has *any* sleeps during the day but is still not tired when he goes to bed at eight (and that was *my* suggestion in Chapter Three) and he sits there sucking a thumb and staring vacantly into space, then you've a rare one indeed. I suspect his bed is too sterile—by that I mean no cuddly animals (companions) in it, no pictures on the wall for him to look at. I am not recommending he be given toys at night-time—construction kits and farmyards, etc. But the odd friend to talk to drowsily, that's different.

Masturbation

Many babies (especially boys) discover that fingering their genitals brings a pleasant sensation, and as they get to two or three they will tend to do it to comfort themselves when they're tired or ill. I'm relieved to say that the Victorian reaction to masturbation—an unpardonable sin, 'cured' by canings, absurd threats that it will drive one mad, or by tying the hands to the bedhead—has passed. Now most mothers realise that any sort of punishment could make a child ashamed of his sexual organs, which could in turn one day distort his attitude to sex.

However, this doesn't stop all mothers from being *embarrassed* by the sight of their one-year-old handling his penis in the bath. I've heard other child experts say that, if you come into this category, it is perfectly all right to divert your infant's attention—pass him his boat to play with, for instance. I quarrel with this advice. If on every occasion when your child begins to masturbate, you immediately urge him to stop (however subtly), he'll very soon know that this is something of which Mummy disapproves. So personally, I would say to embarrassed mums : find something to divert *your own* attention. Polish the taps of the wash-hand basin or something, until he's finished.

By the time your child has outgrown babyhood, masturbation will instinctively have become a private thing, confined to his bed—because that's where he is when he's sleepy or sick, isn't it? And should your four- or five-year-old start doing it in the living-room, without any comment or indication of censure, take him to his bed. In this way he'll absorb the idea that whilst masturbation isn't terrible or wrong, it is not something that is socially acceptable in public.

Finally, I would add that if this habit becomes excessive in your opinion, your child is probably emotionally disturbed and you should consult a paediatrician.

Nose-picking

A really horrible one, this. I have a theory that it starts after a cold (and one- to five-year-olds have an awful lot of colds) when the mucous dries up and forms annoying 'bogies' in the nostrils. The child removes them with his finger and finds to his satisfaction that this stops the irritation. And from that moment on, his mother will be saying : 'Not your finger, dear; use a tissue . . .'

So to follow through logically : if whenever you wash your child's face, you check that his nose is clean, too, the desire to nose-pick should never arise.

For babies and toddlers, cotton-wool buds are ideal for nose-care. (Or so my daughter tells me—actually I get on better with a tissue.) For later on, I would suggest you have a box of clean tissues in every key room in the house, because 'up in the front bedroom' can seem a long way away to a child with a picking-finger poised. Nose hygiene should also prevent that other ghastly habit : sniffing.

Nail-biting

I ought to confess right away that I was a nail-biter myself. My mother tried everything under the sun to stop me, and no method succeeded. But where a mother may fail over some thirteen years, a first love succeeds in a couple of meetings ! There I was, in romantic pre-war Vienna, fifteen years old and wildly in love with a blond and handsome Austrian. I shall never forget it : he lifted my hand to his lips to kiss, he held my bitten-away fingernails—and quietly put my hand down again . . . without the kiss. I never bit my nails again after that day.

Still, for parents who are not prepared to wait thirteen years for a cure, the best idea I've heard is to say nothing when you notice your small child nibbling at his fingernails, but at wash-time paint on a substance like 'Stop and Grow'. Tell him chattily that it's to make his nails look pretty, and put some on your own to prove the point. Then pray. If you're lucky, the next time he puts his fingers into his mouth, the nasty taste will put him off for life. He must never, however, suspect that you engineered the whole thing.

Be prepared for failure, though. Determined nail-biters can even acquire a taste for Bitter Aloes. I know, because my younger daughter did! I've used every argument on Merle my mother used on me, and none of them stopped her. What eventually did the trick—you've guessed it—was vanity and a boy friend.

Nervous habits

There are hundreds of annoying little habits that children can adopt—from twitching at an ear to wiggling a piece of string. I think it's all right to mention it once, or even twice. 'Look, do you suppose your ear enjoys being pulled like that? If I were your ear, I wouldn't . . .' Sometimes, just being aware one has a certain gesture is sufficient to enable one to control it.

But treat it lightly. And if at all possible, unobtrusively find the offending hand or whatever something more constructive to do. Never nag about it or continually draw attention to it; that only makes it worse. It's like the smoker who needs a cigarette to fiddle with. Should you ask him *why* he wants something in his hand, he'll become more aware of his idle fingers, not less.

You may regard some habit your child has as really anti-social and deserving of smacks; well, that's your decision as a parent. But I have a hunch punishment won't help. I believe there are some people who need a footling physical activity to offset the mental activity of concentration—whether it's the four-year-old playing dolls or an adult like Patricia, who during the gruelling editing of this book chewed five whole pencils to death!

CHAPTER TEN

Your Child and Other Animals

You will be aware, of course, that this title is cribbed quite blatantly from Gerald Durrell, a man I know and admire very much. In our case the chapter title refers to your child in relationship to *your* friends, your child in relationship to his own friends; and finally, in truth, your child in relationship to animals—the four-legged kind, the furry kind, both your own and other people's.

Your friends
Let me say right away that there is no reason why your friends, even your closest friends, should be as enamoured of your child as you are, and vice versa. I had a dear friend who was like a sister to me, but my elder daughter, then about six months old, disliked her intensely and screamed loudly whenever she came near. Since Tina had seen the friend frequently before and nothing about her appearance or manner had changed and could be frightening her, we came to the conclusion that for one reason or another my baby didn't like my friend. After that, my friend, being a very sensible woman, kept at a respectful distance. There was no more picking the baby up and cuddling her; in fact she ignored Tina. And there was no more trouble. Peace reigned, and no one was upset. I certainly wasn't; my friend wasn't; and Tina was downright relieved. So if a baby can take exception to a particular person for some reason all her own, how much more can a four-year-old have a special—to you, unfounded—dislike?

That's fair enough. But it doesn't mean your child should

166

be permitted to behave rudely or be insulting. He may come out with bald statements such as 'I don't like you' anyway; but if he does, he should be reprimanded because hurting visitors' feelings is unkind and inhospitable. Parents should always insist their children are as polite and as well behaved towards their friends as their age allows. They should say 'hello', 'goodbye', 'please', 'thank you' and the normal things which oil the wheels of social relationships. Good gracious, your child is probably going to dislike somebody one day much more than your friend Marjorie, someone he's *got* to be polite to—his history master, his boss, his sister-in-law, so he might as well get used to the conventions now. So we can demand polite behaviour but we cannot enforce (and we shouldn't attempt to) a loving relationship where no love exists.

You will also have friends who, although they may be very charming people themselves, just don't like young children. They possibly haven't children of their own or perhaps, dreadful thought, they may dislike your particular child. I occasionally find that people whom I personally like very much have children whom I have very little time for—children not reared in the discipline tradition of *The New Childhood*! Yet I still like the parents as social contacts for me. Come to that, over the years we have made many friends who hadn't the slightest interest in *our* children.

The point is: if friends seem uncomfortable in your child's presence, my advice is not to try and 'convert' them by putting your little girl in a pretty, frilly dress and lecturing her on 'manners', but just to accept that we all have our personal preferences. Whilst I don't think you ought to make your daughter vanish, by banning her from the living-room, you most certainly can avoid thrusting her down their throats. Don't let her pester them to play with her (that goes for the most sentimental child-lover too: only the guest who *really wants to* should be let in for reading a story), and watch what *you* do with her in front of them. Don't change her nappy in the room where they're sitting. Don't eat up the soggy remnants of her tea. These are the sort of actions that can put your friends off you, and children in general, for ever.

By the way, I think it is unneccessary for every acquaintance to be called 'Auntie' or 'Uncle'. If you yourself are on first-name terms with somebody, surely now, in the twentieth century, it is perfectly polite for your children also to address them as 'Jean' or 'Peter' or whatever their name is? If Jean and Peter themselves object, that's different. But to my way of thinking, 'Auntie' and 'Uncle' should be reserved for relations.

Children under five often cannot understand intellectually who is and who is not a member of the family. I have seen considerable confusion arise over who is a proper auntie and who is not a proper auntie, or a real uncle, and I suppose the alternative there is an unreal uncle! So for friend Peter: 'Peter' if possible, even 'Mr Brugenheimer' but not 'Uncle Peter'. Incidentally, when visiting Jean and Peter for a day cum evening, I recommend putting your child to bed in their house, at his usual bedtime with his usual ritual: bath, pyjamas, Teddy, etc. Then at 11 or 12 p.m., all you need do is carry sleepy child in thick blanket out to the car (and a car is an essential here) and simply lift him into his own bed once you're home. It avoids both curtailing your evening and getting your child overtired.

Just one final appeal to make before we leave the subject of your friends: never, never, never discuss your child with them in the child's hearing. Praise will make him precocious and vain; criticism will make him feel inferior and betrayed; and simply talking about him will make him self-conscious. General conversation which includes the child ('We went to the zoo yesterday, and Johnnie had a ride on the elephant—didn't you, Johnnie . . .') that's different and beneficial. But discussing *him* ('Johnnie started nursery school last week and he seemed shy of the other children . . .') that's unforgiveable.

I often meet mothers in the street whose children I helped deliver. 'Look, Matthew,' they say, 'this is the lady who brought you into the world.' I can positively see poor Matthew squirm with embarrassment—because he's being made an *object* for discussion. Then blessedly, Mother passes on to the weather, her holiday, Grandpa's bronchitis, and all the ordinary grown-ups' chat; and Matthew, though bored stiff, can at least relax.

I would add that children find adult conversation awfully dull. As a five-year-old myself I was made to suffer interminable teas at which I had to be seen but I was never allowed to be heard. I used to go home positively bursting to say something. So on behalf of the current generation of young children, may I request that when they say, 'Mummy . . .' and you say, 'Just a moment, dear; Jean's speaking . . .', you remember them *in a moment*. When Jean has finished her sentence, you should turn to your small son or daughter and ask pleasantly and attentively, what it is he or she wants to say.

Your child's friends

Just as your child and your friends may not be the best of chums, there is also no reason to suppose that your child and your friends' children will be bosom pals. I know of many instances where the children loathe the sight of each other but are nevertheless forced to spend many boring Sundays in one another's company because the parents wish to spend the day together. As a result, the children become nasty, irritable and fretful. It would be vastly preferable if these Sunday visits were cut down to a minimum and instead the parents met when their children weren't around—in the evening, say. The trouble is: many parents are not aware of the fact that two three-year-olds do not necessarily make two close friends, any more than two brothers make two intimates. Put any child into a nursery school, or later into the Infants, and he'll become best friends, not with the whole class, but with somebody.

Now, obviously, his teacher will insist on politeness towards everybody in the class, may he like the individual concerned or may he not, but no teacher would dream of insisting on an intimate friendship between two children. Teachers know that friendship will develop only if the two children want it. So take a leaf out of Teacher's book: politeness to everybody, but friendship only where your child chooses.

And once your child has made a choice, almost inevitably you get a 'She's my best friend; I hate her' situation. Your three to five-year-old child begins to have squabbles and rows and scenes, not with you—not the wilful defiance of Mother, which the two and three-year-olds are so good at—but with his or her own 'friends'. Your child comes to you and complains that whoever it was hit him or whoever it was took his favourite ball, doll, car. What do you do? Firstly, play it by ear.

I think it is extremely unwise to get involved in every squabble your child has, because it is only too easy to wind up an enemy of every child's parents with whom he has ever played! Children fight about something and they hate each other. It doesn't last long—the next day, sometimes the next minute, they're best friends again. Not so the adults who champion them. Criticise someone's darling child and a grudge may be borne against you for life! So wherever possible, let your child fight his own battles, settle his own scores.

Occasionally, of course, you have to get involved. If there is physical injury (and that means injury inflicted by either side —your child is no more an angel than any other child), if he's been bashed by somebody and somebody else has a black eye, then this ought to be acknowledged and amends made. A lecture, an apology, even a punishment: you should take whatever steps are required. If you need to claim back a toy, an expensive toy perhaps, which you feel your child ought to keep, visit the other child's parents on a 'What can we adults do together about this disagreement between our children?' basis, rather than an accusatory one: 'Your child has taken Tracy's doll's pram; what are you going to do about it?' The desire to defend one's young is very strong in all of us, and so be on your guard not to provoke it in your neighbour. It isn't fair that you should have to become isolated in a community just because your child is still learning about the give-and-take of human relationships.

How can you assist your child in learning this? Only, I fear, by example. The rest he'll have to find out the hard way: for himself. I mean, if a four-year-old's so bossy other children refuse to play with him, it is to be hoped that in the ensuing loneliness he'll realise the error of his ways and the next week be a little more tentative when he joins in the game. The same goes for the spiteful child, or the one who won't share his toys. If you notice an anti-social trait in your own child, of course you can try pointing it out to him. But do-as-you-would-be-done-by as a philosophy ('How would you like it if Adam never let you have a turn on the tricycle?') is awfully sophisticated for an under-five to follow. He can't imagine himself in Adam's shoes, standing on the grass, and Adam becoming him racing away on the tricycle. It's all too complicated.

Example is what counts in the long run. He will be considerate to other children if his parents are considerate to him. It isn't any good trying to stop your child hitting and shouting if you yourself are given to sudden outbursts, during which you whack and bellow, and all the doors and windows rattle. Your child will also lose his temper and bellow, because this is obviously the standard you expect in your house—whatever you may say to the contrary.

As we've said before : friendships for your child are absolutely essential. However, he's bound to make some friends with whom, for various reasons, you'd prefer him not to associate. Remain cool; don't break up the acquaintance. The more force you apply, the more you forbid the association, the more resistance you will create in your child. (I've often thought that if the Montagues and Capulets hadn't opposed the match so violently, Romeo and Juliet might well have drifted apart!) In any case, it isn't necessary to part him from some young friend he values. Providing your child's home is a happy one and the standards there consistently high, your influence will prevail over anyone's else's, especially another three or four-year-old's.

Pets

There is a theory that it is good for children to have pets to look after. It's true, but it doesn't apply to under-five-year-olds. Certainly it is still beneficial for them to live with animals in the house, but don't imagine that the puppy you give your child for Christmas will be looked after by him. (Personally, I object to an animal belonging to a particular member of the family anyway, because by virtue of the fact that it lives with the family, it will be fed, cleaned, exercised and played with by everyone.) A child under five isn't capable of undertaking that responsibility. You still have to buy the food; you still have to see that the dog's bedding is washed; you still have to groom it, although the child can help. He can't go off and walk the dog for an hour—not under the age of five. If the pet's been involved in a fight, *you* have to deal with the wound;

if it has pups, *you* have to call the vet and later advertise for owners. You can't expect the young child whose puppy it originally was, because somebody gave it to him as a present, to attain the necessary wisdom overnight.

So to all those people who believe their child needs a pet, I would ask : do you yourselves want one?—because it's going to mean a lot of drudgery for you, not him. If the answer's yes, then a dog or a cat and, to a lesser extent, a guinea pig, goldfish, budgerigar, rabbit or a dozen other similar household animals are excellent for your child. Apart from providing companionship and entertainment, they will begin to teach him that someone else can depend on him. Remembering that 'Spot' needs his dinner or that 'Mitzi' the long-haired Guinea Pig ought to be combed will develop a sense of responsibility in your child, not to mention bringing out such virtues in him as kindness, unselfishness and gentleness.

Granted, some authorities may claim that young children living in close proximity with animals is unhygienic, and they are possibly right. I can only reply that my cat, my dog and my children all slept very happily in the same room—even, I suspect, at times on the same bed—for several years, and nothing dreadful, traumatic or otherwise unfortunate happened to any of them as a result. I admit that I couldn't always stop the dog licking the three-year-old's face but then Souha always took her duties seriously. On one memorable occasion my toddler decided to share a matey dog biscuit with Souha; yet I'm still convinced the advantages of having pets outweigh the slight risk of infection. One thing : my children all grew up fearless of animals. None of them ever dreaded a walk to the shops in case he should encounter a strange dog on the way, and that in itself is quite a boon.

If anything, I did a little too well in that direction. I once spent a weary two hours sitting in a local hospital with Merle waiting for an anti-tetanus injection. She had picked up a stray kitten, which in fright had ripped a piece of skin off her wrist. It wasn't her fault; on the contrary, she'd held the kitten the way we'd taught her. But nervous and unused to humans, it had scratched her in its attempt to escape. So here endeth the first lesson : warn your child that strange animals

are not necessarily as friendly as your own. Tell him never to
approach a pet (especially a dog) he doesn't know without
first making sure it is willing to be favoured. Show him how
to offer the back of his hand for the dog to smell and accept, before he attempts to pat it. And if the dog is growling and jumping furiously, not to go up to it at all but to give it a wide berth.

And having decided to get a dog or cat, you come to the
controversy of when is the best age from your child's view-
point. (If you already own a dog before you have your family,
this question won't arise. You're unlikely to delay starting a baby
for five years to accommodate your pet!) I would say definitely not within the first nine months. At this stage perfect
hygiene is so vital (you should not have a crawling baby with
an un-house-trained pup), and you have enough work what
with the nappies and the 6 a.m. feed without taking on any
more.

My husband and I waited until Merle was two (and Tina,
incidentally, eight) before we had Souha—a six-week-old
shaggy sheepdog pup. And let me tell you : having two tots in
the household (one two-legged and the other four-legged) is
a fine song and dance. Typical of all young animals, Merle
and Souha fought dozens of times a day. The puppy would
grip the child's ankle sock with its teeth and hold on. Screams
from child. My husband Ian or I would rush and separate
them, only to find two minutes later that the child had now
grasped the puppy's tail in her fist. Yelps from puppy. However many times we separated them, however many times we
punished the one who was inflicting the injury at the time,
they always came together again. We couldn't turn our backs
for five minutes. Then finally we found a simple expedient :
every time there was a yelp from one or a scream from the
other, we smacked both regardless—the hand and the snout.
Like the warring brother and sister we discussed in Chapter
Three, puppy and toddler soon learnt that telling tales only
got them both into trouble. Within a week they were the
best of friends, and in fact they never attacked each other
again. So if you feel strong enough to buy a kitten or puppy
while your child is still under three, I recommend you to try the
same method of keeping the peace.

There's one thing to be said for putting up with a puppy and a toddler simultaneously : you get your reward when the next baby comes along. By then the dog is an adult. It's always lived with a child and so it isn't jealous of the new arrival; in fact, it is very often protective.

In our case Souha was just over a year when Nicholas was born. She had watched our preparations for the new baby for many weeks, had looked curiously at the carry-cot which was waiting all ready, and finally had seen the baby lying in it. Nicholas was actually born in hospital but we came home within forty-eight hours. And on that first morning, when the district midwife came to attend me and bath the baby, something odd happened. The cot was on its stand between my bed and the wall; but when the midwife tried to slide the cot out, it wouldn't move. It appeared to be stuck. As she tugged and pulled, I glanced down—and saw Souha, usually a friendly, docile dog, lying right across the legs of the stand with her teeth bared a couple of inches from the midwife's ankle! Believing that occasionally discretion is the better part of valour, I instructed the midwife to retreat and then passed the baby out to her; it seemed wiser than disturbing a guard on duty.

From that morning Souha was the best nanny I could have had. When the baby was out in his pram, the dog sat beside it, on constant alert. If Nicholas so much as whimpered, in came Souha and nudged my leg until I went out to see what was wrong. I might add that no cat was foolish enough to venture within sight! And later on, the dog bore all sorts of pokings and pullings from Nicholas without a snarl; the most she ever did in the way of protest was to walk away.

So a young fully-grown dog, between two and five, is probably the ideal with an infant. If you can't bear the pup idea, you could always take on someone else's older pet, perhaps through the R.S.P.C.A. or a dogs' home.

What I would guard against is acquiring an old dog which has been totally unused to the wear and tear of young children. It might well be a little tetchy about the however unintentional rough handling it receives. And when that happens, a pet is more of a worry than a joy.

Generally speaking, though, animals enrich a child's life, which is why a visit, or better still, a holiday, at a farm is so valuable. It always seems to me a lack that modern town children hardly know what cows, sheep, horses, pigs, donkeys, chicken, geese and so forth look like, except from picture-books and on television. Living on a farm for a while and getting close to animals : watching them sleep, feed, being shorn, cared for; seeing horses groomed, cows milked, having a ride on a donkey . . . they are all a part of the ever-widening experience of life.

CHAPTER ELEVEN

It's a Date!

EVERY so often in family life there are special occasions—dates you note down in your diary and plan for weeks ahead. In my opinion some of these dates should include your child (in the case of his birthday, for instance, the celebration would be a little pointless without him!) but equally some of them shouldn't. Personally I feel that children under five do not belong at a relation's wedding reception buffet, at their grandparents' twenty-fifth Wedding Anniversary luncheon or at a young aunt's engagement party. They get in the way, turning what should have been a 'treat day' for you into a nightmare of 'don't touch', 'Susie, where are you?', 'Johnnie, you can't play "He" round the cake.' So don't drag your child along to get bored, frustrated and upset; leave him at home with a sitter.

And on the subject of weddings, think twice about being flattered into letting your little girl be a bridesmaid. It's the six to ten-year-olds who adore the long dresses and all the fuss, not our age-group. The two, three or four-year-old will at best be over-excited by all the attention; at worst she'll howl.

However, there are family gatherings where the children are an integral part: for example, a Golden Wedding Day when the elderly couple invite their score of descendents to tea. On such an occasion there would be the sort of food children could enjoy, other youngsters to play with, and plenty of benign adults around to supervise. Christmas is a similar time. But possibly the very first date in your child's social diary is rather different: his Christening.

o – 1 year

CHRISTENING

I must say right away that I'm a firm believer in total religious
freedom. I am certainly not suggesting that because your
Faith may have no baptism ceremony or because you feel
christening is stuff and nonsense, you are automatically found
wanting as a good parent. It is not my business either to
advocate or condemn christening in principle; but for the sake
of the majority of people in this country who do have their
children christened, it would be shirking the issue if I didn't
comment on this event at all.

Now, it occurs to me that the religious service and the social
gathering of a baby's christening have become almost insepar-
able, and I fear this is not a good thing. The Victorian photo-
graph of Mama gliding down the staircase in her trailing
dress carrying the new baby in his best robe may have looked
all very fine; but do let's remember that she had a bevy of
servants to help her with all the preparations, and a Nanny
standing by to remove the infant at the auspicious moment.
Nowadays, when we do our own catering and can't possibly
consider employing a Nanny, the hostess bit comes a trifle hard
when one is getting up at 2 a.m. for the night-feed and still
hasn't quite mastered that daily schedule the pamphlet listed so
glibly. And if the baby is only weeks old, then the mother
will probably not have recovered her full physical energy yet,
either.

When I suggested to a young mum that giving an enormous
party within two months of childbirth was perhaps rash,
she said in a shocked voice : 'But the party's not for *my* benefit;
it's for the baby's!'

H'mmm, is it? I have yet to meet the baby who enjoyed his
christening party. In my experience every one has found it
upsetting. Stands to reason, doesn't it? The baby's routine
is interfered with. Lunch comes up early because he has to be
at the church by 3 o'clock; his afternoon rest doesn't materialise
for hours; and tea is late because Mother has to be with her
guests for the champagne toast. There are strange people about,
people making a lot of noise and maybe smoking . . . and, most
objectionable of all, peering at him. And finally, if the baby is

being breast-fed, he won't appreciate the decrease in his milk supply due to his mother's nervous tension and tiredness.

But aren't we somewhat stuck with the christening in its present form? No, say I, not if we've a mind to rebel. If it's a question of aunts and friends wanting 'to see the baby', I advise that you invite them round in twos and threes for a simple cup of tea. In this way they and the baby will have a chance to become properly acquainted as individuals instead of a horde. I realise that a daytime get-together generally has to exclude the menfolk; but it takes a very exceptional man to want to hold and talk to a new baby—someone else's new baby, that is. Usually, a quick glance in the cot when he pops round for a cards evening will satisfy him!

As for the christening ceremony . . . Well, you don't *need* dozens of onlookers there either—just the three of you, the three godparents (the C of E tradition is two god*fathers* and one god*mother* for a boy, and vice versa for a girl) and possibly the grandparents. Which I count as a mere ten for whom the young mother will have to serve tea. And your child does not have to be christened while still a babe-in-arms, anyway. Whilst I have the greatest respect for people who wish to commit their child to the christian faith officially, in church, as soon as possible, I am wary of those who do it as a matter of form—a job to get through: 'because it could be embarrassing for him later if he isn't "done" now'.

In fact my own eldest wasn't christened until she was four, and I think she benefitted from the delay. Tina attended Sunday school and, on learning that all the other boys and girls there had apparently been 'christened', she asked to be christened, too. Because she was both old enough to understand what was going on and also because it was by her own choice, the service meant a great deal more to her. Moreover, the teachers there used the service to demonstrate the religious meaning of christening to the rest of the Sunday school. Three of those teachers, incidentally, acted as godparents.

Ian and I had plenty of friends, good, loyal friends who would have undertaken the task if we'd asked them. But we considered what those godparents had to promise, and then we asked ourselves frankly whether we'd resent it if those Easter-Christmas-weddings-and-funerals church friends of ours one day called round to criticise our spiritual upbringing of Tina. The answer was 'yes' we would, which would have made nonsense of their role. So we selected instead these three dedicated Christians, who indeed carried out their duties admirably, even helping us find a Church-of-England school for Tina.

Perhaps we carried things to extremes, but I think we were right in principle.

BIRTHDAYS

The next big occasion in your child's calendar is his first birthday.

Yes, I know there is a tradition among many young parents to make much of their offspring's first birthday. They prepare a fancy tea; they buy a cake with one candle on it; they invite other children of his or her age, along with *their mothers*...

Do you seriously imagine that a one-year-old, who has absolutely no ability to integrate socially with people of his own age, enjoys such a party? If he feels amenable that day, he might accept it; but if he's tired or crotchety or teething, then he's going to be upset by all the strangeness, by the highly-suspect presence of these other babies, and by his mother's preoccupation with the entertaining. Thus the person who least enjoys his birthday is himself. All his parents have achieved is to have carried on the social tradition in their circle, and that's not what parents are for, is it?

How much better for your family to break away and celebrate the day quietly. There is so much time (a whole lifetime) for big, noisy parties, when your child will be able to handle his role as host; but he's not ready for those parties yet. So this year let him spend it just with you, Father if at all possible, and his older brothers and sisters, who, for once, should be encouraged to put themselves out for the birthday child. As for the other three or four guests: they should be *his* friends—adults with endless patience for Peepbo, ball rolling, knee bouncing and a host of other splendid pastimes.

And believe me: your baby's tummy is far safer with the odd treat, like chocolate biscuit instead of bread-and-jam and ice-cream instead of a piece of apple, than with a whole table full of 'birthday tea'. Moreover, he'd rather have you playing with him on the floor than dashing about being a good hostess.

I've said it a dozen times: the young child needs time to appreciate things—the candle on his cake, a new toy he's been given (and I'd suggest you space out his presents; a whole mass will only confuse him) and his pretty cards. Incidentally, if you've the sort of child who genuinely likes looking at pictures and carting them about, then I'd allow him to play with his birthday cards. After all, they were sent for his pleasure, not just to be displayed proudly on the mantelpiece.

1 – 2 years

Almost all of what I've just said applies equally to Birthday two. By now your child may well appreciate companions of his own age, but I doubt if he'll welcome his sparring partners on *his* day. Much as he'd miss these friends of his if he couldn't play with them ordinarily, I suspect his idea of bliss is to have all his new toys to himself, the undistracted attention of Mother, and a favourite tea in his own chair. Two-year-olds, remember, are famous for their tantrums; in a party tea atmosphere you're bound to spark off at least one of them, probably the small host.

2 – 3 years

All right: I'll give you this one. On his third birthday your child might indeed enjoy having a small party. He won't like forty small guests (thank heaven); he won't even like fourteen; but around a half-dozen other children between three and five will probably please him a lot. Invite children he likes and knows well; otherwise shyness or tears may strike and the party will be ruined. So ask his young cousin, the little boy across the road, a friend's daughter with whom he always plays happily and, if he attends one yet, his closest pals from Playgroup. Unless you help there yourself, you may have to ask the Playgroup Leader who those pals are, because children under five are notorious for never mentioning Best Friend Simon's existence. And needless to say: *you* speak to Simon's mother. If you leave it to the lads, Simon will either come back that same day or else never at all!

By the way, a delightful birthday idea for children who attend Playgroup or Nursery Class in the afternoons, is to hold the celebration at teatime at school. *You* provide the sandwiches and cake and the balloons and whistles and so on; but the teacher, with the experience, retains control. It's an excellent compromise, because it means that you share the festivity with your child without being worried about dealing with the mechanics of the party. What's more, his guests are all the small people with whom he's learning to form relationships on a regular basis. One other advantage: it avoids the necessity of having lots of other mothers around.

If you do have to have the party at home (and presumably even though he has this birthday tea at nursery school, he will want some sort of celebration with his family), do watch that the adults around don't take over the day. I appreciate that many three-year-olds cannot adjust happily to unfamiliar surroundings unless their mothers are there, and so you may have to invite some parents. Just be sure that the occasion remains 'child-orientated'. In other words, the action is centred round the children's pleasure and doesn't drift into a natter-session or cocktail-party for the mums.

3 – 5 years

For the fourth birthday and finally for the fifth, I'd make a rule: 'no mothers'. By now your child will want around ten guests at his party, and that's quite enough without ten adults as well. Granted, you're going to need help; but I think it's better if your ally both Behind the Lines in the kitchen and at the Front in the games room, isn't one of the other children's mothers because he is likely to be embarrassed by her presence and show off, which will *add* to your trouble, not lessen it.

Naturally, Father is the perfect choice . . . but only if Father honestly wants to be there. From experience we all know that most fathers, however devoted otherwise, however keen on their child's upbringing, however willing to participate in his practical day-to-day care, heartily dislike small children's tea parties. So if you're not lucky enough to be married to one of the rare saints, give in gracefully. Take it from one who knows. There is no point in bringing pressure to bear on a reluctant man to organise Musical Bumps. If your husband shudders at the very idea, he is honestly better off out of the way. You and your friend will get on faster without him.

Doing what? Supervising tea and organising, organising, organising. If your party invitations state '*from 3 o'clock till six*', allow forty minutes for tea and fill the majority of the rest of the time with organised games. If you're fortunate enough to have a garden with play equipment in it—sand-pit, paddling pool, swing, climbing-frame, tent, tricycle, a lawn large enough for ball games, you're away, if the birthday is in the summer. All you will have to do is be around with a beady eye and a first-aid kit. But if your party is to be held indoors, and you leave the children to amuse themselves, anarchy will reign. They need to be told what to do; they need the security of knowing someone bigger than they is in charge.

There are a number of books on the market which describe games suitable for different age-groups, including three to five-year-olds. But if their suggestions don't inspire you greatly, perhaps the best people to consult would be the local nursery school teacher or Playgroup leader, because these people have first-hand knowledge of what children genuinely like to play. There are certain basic favourites, but I think every party should have at least one original game as well. Whatever is played, though, keep it simple. I've seen adults with high I.Q.s utterly baffled by the rules of a new game as described by their hostess (and three other people simultaneously); so take pity on an under-five.

And do remember that the attention-span of three to five-year-olds is short. Almost any game which lasts longer than ten minutes should be discarded before you begin, because a percentage of your guests will become bored by it and will not continue to participate. You will then have a little rival faction amusing itself while you are desperately trying to maintain the official entertainment. This can also happen with elimination games—the ones who are OUT grow bored just watching. *Before* they begin jumping from chair to chair, see that your second adult is keeping them busy.

If you decide to award prizes for the games, then it is your job as the host's adult representative to ensure than every child wins something. The child whose pin comes nearest to the donkey is an undisputed winner, but it's mighty easy to 'fix' Pass the Parcel or Musical Chairs so that the winner is someone different. Bend backwards and sideways to make sure that no child, including your own, is left out. I know your own child has already received 'X' number of presents, but a prize is a perk—something to be proud of.

All children love to have something to show off at home. So even if you don't agree with 'prizes', I fear you'll have to distribute loot. These take-home gifts needn't be expensive— wax crayons, a plastic car, or even just a balloon. But make much of the giving. Have the gifts drawn from a bran tub, or handed out by a dressed-up Santa Claus (if the party occurs around the Christmas season). I'm well aware that even tiny presents add to the financial burden of the party; but I'm afraid they help it to be judged a success by the children.

As for The Tea: veteran party-givers tell me that one should Think Disposable and do away with the washing-up. These days the designs on paper beakers, plates, napkins, etc., are so attractive they look almost nicer than the real thing anyway. And if you're holding the party at nursery school or in a hired hut, throw-away crockery does solve a tricky transport problem.

With regard to the food itself, always bear in mind that young children are the most conservative of eaters. 'What's *that*?' they say, turning up their noses at anything unfamiliar. So now is not the time to present an avocado salad! What I've found goes down well is familiar foods in unfamiliar guises, and savouries at that. Things on cocktail-sticks are popular because they're offered in small amounts—sausages, cubes of cheese and pineapple, pieces of ham. Another good idea is cracker biscuits, thinly spread with butter, with cheese or chicken on top. And in summer nothing is more appetising than a dish of red baby tomatoes which a child can pop in his mouth whole, or scrubbed new carrots—the miniature kind you buy in bunches. And a platter of potato crisps, Twiglets and salted peanuts will most assuredly vanish.

Passing on to the next course as it were . . . ice-cream is a Must. And almost all children in our age-group like jelly; so it helps if the jelly is in individual trifle cups ready. It's one less serving job to do during the devouring session. If you think jelly on its own is a bit dull—and I must confess I do—add fresh or tinned fruit. Beware, though, of doing something clever with the biscuits. In the past I've spent an hour baking home-made coconut creams, only to have them regarded with sus-picion by Merle's friends, and finally to be asked for the shop-bought packet they recognised!

And to drink, I don't think you can better squashes. Yes, I know I said I wasn't in favour of them; but this is a *birthday*, for heaven's sake!

And lastly we come to the Ceremonial Birthday Cake. But by now nearly all the children will be too full up to eat any and, besides, many of them find the traditional marzipaned and white-iced cake far too rich. That's why I'd go for a chocolate sponge with cream in it instead. The candles—to be blown out to a rousing chorus of 'Happy Birthday'—look just as good on that. But if you really do fancy an iced birthday cake, be prepared to wrap the pieces in napkins ready for your small guests to take home to their mothers.

Before I leave food, let me issue a warning. Children don't eat a quarter of what you assume they will. Don't over-cater; it will break your heart.

Ending a party is as difficult as starting one. You don't want to have the children just sitting around, bored, waiting to be collected. And on the other hand, it's unfair to play a wildly stimulating game from which their mothers will have to drag them away. If your budget will run to it, the ideal is a hired conjuror or ventriloquist for quarter of an hour : or if you have a movie projector, a short cartoon film. But if these ideas are far too extravagant, then a fitting end to a very nice day would be to read a story from a new book your child's been given. Once again, your extra adult is valuable : because if she's reading the story, then you're free to answer the door to the mothers and perhaps give them a cup of tea.

And at the actual moment of parting, your child should be taught the social graces of saying 'Thank you for coming to my party', just as his guest should say 'Thank you for having me'. Incidentally, when your child is a *guest* at a party, don't ever humiliate him by arriving late to collect him. If the invitation said '6 *o'clock*', be there at six, having allowed for the traffic jam or missing the bus. Don't make him sit there all alone looking spare.

CHRISTMAS

Christmas with children in the house is wonderful. At the risk of sounding sentimental for once, the peaceful, gourmet, sophisticated Christmases my family enjoys now are certainly not as exhausting as they used to be; but they're not as much fun, not as magic somehow either. So appreciate this decade or so of family Christmases, tiring though they are, while you may; they won't last forever. But don't imagine they *start* the moment you have a baby.

0 – 18 months

I've said it time and time again: babies like familiarity and routine—and the 24th, 25th and 26th of December are to them just three more days. Certainly with the baby under a year, you should aim to keep the part of the day when he's up and about as quiet and close to an ordinary Saturday as possible. Even when he's over a year, take it gently. He can't comprehend what Christmas is all about, and the tense excitement and noise could easily distress him. And don't be surprised if he plays with the fancy wrappings and the boxes with great glee, but ignores his presents which were contained inside. That's typical!

By all means give your child a turkey dinner in gravy with potato and perhaps two or three sprouts; but lay off the cranberry jelly and the leeks and the Xmas pudding; or he'll pay you back by crying all evening with stomach-ache, when you're entertaining friends to supper or trying to watch the best movie they've had on TV in years!

18 months – 5 years

As your child grows out of babyhood, Christmas becomes a day
on which things are exciting although he doesn't quite understand why they are exciting. He knows only that it's something
to look forward to. He knows the day is nearing when Mother
brings in a Christmas tree and hangs it with coloured lights
and bubbles and tinsel to make it bright and pretty. (Even a
young baby will watch the lights flickering on and off.)

But its very attraction spells danger to a young child. Unless
it is behind a fixed fireguard or high enough up so that it is
out of reach, your child may well grasp one of the glass balls
and hurt himself—or pull the whole tree over and hurt you
. . . if not so physically. And, of course, never be tempted to use
lighted candles however graceful and enchanting they may look
—the fire risk just isn't worth the candle !

I'm against letting a child under five help hang the decora-
tions, both on the tree and round the room, because it's a long
job (it always takes us hours longer than we allow) and he'll
soon get very bored. He'll do things with the sticky-tape you
asked him to hold and the holly-berries lying on the floor, you
hadn't intended him to do at all; and he'll play with the scissors
and empty the pin-box . . . And you'll wind up cursing Christmas, your child and any merry gentleman who is foolish
enough to put his head round the door !

So I would suggest you decorate after your child is asleep in
bed, and then watch the delight on his face next morning when
he comes down to find the lounge transformed into fairyland.

At midnight on Christmas Eve Father Christmas comes.
Now I know an argument rages that he is nothing to do with
the birth of Christ, that pretending he exists is telling your
child a lie, that accepting the jovial figure on Christmas cards
is commercialising and debasing Christmas . . . Well, the
people who say those things may well be correct. But *I* like
Father Christmas, and I think he adds to the festive spirit. In
our family he always left a stocking at the foot of the bed and
drank the milk the children left out for him. The stockings
contained titbits only—a doll's-house bed, a bar of chocolate,
crayons, a Matchbox car, a tangerine, a yo-yo—but those titbits were a heap of bounty to a waking child.

After breakfast they were allowed to unwrap all the presents sent by friends who would not be spending the holiday with us. These were quite definitely from Jean and Peter or Mr and Mrs Bloggs, and not from Father Christmas. We explained that this was the Season of Goodwill and people express their goodwill towards each other by giving presents. At the same time this system got round the awkward one of Mr and Mrs B. expecting to be thanked for their gifts and the child not appreciating it was from them. Then from unwrapping time till lunch, I do not think it's unreasonable for any child to play with his new toys or his old Dad while Mother gets on with her cooking.

After lunch in our home came the big ceremony of family present-giving. These were either handed round by the youngest children or by 'Father Christmas', some well-intentioned male friend who had been persuaded or bribed to don a dressing-gown covered in red paper and a white cotton-wool beard and carry a sack loaded with gifts. If the children half-recognised Uncle Tom, they didn't let on. In fact my children told me only recently how they kept it from us for a couple of years that they no longer believed in Father Christmas. They thought we'd be disappointed. They were right. It was fun thinking up various ways of hanging those stockings in their rooms without being seen. Christmas never was quite the same without Santa Claus...

Returning to that present-giving ceremony. This is the climax of the day, and in the intense excitement it is not unusual for a young child to fall asleep with exhaustion. Don't forget that he was probably awake late the previous night with excitement and woke early that morning to get to his stocking. Don't rouse him. Put him quietly in his bed and save the rest of his presents (and one belonging to each other child who's there) until he wakes up again.

What those presents should be depends on the individual tastes of your child. But I can suggest a few things they *shouldn't* be. Perhaps if I list some of the mistakes Ian and I and other parents have made, it might save you and your child from disappointment.

A rocking-horse superbly carved and complete with leather

saddle and reins may look very impressive to an adult, but there isn't much a three or four-year-old can use it for. He or she isn't old enough for imaginative cowboy (for boys) and fairytale prince (for girls) games, which require a horse to ride. On the other hand they've outgrown such passive entertainment as mounting this toy and rocking for hours on end.

A similar error is the large beautifully-dressed doll, often Italian. A child will press her nose to the shop-window and beg you to buy it for her. But once she owns it, she finds there's nothing she can do with it *but* admire it . . . and she could have done that much from outside the shop. She can't wash its clothes; she can't pin up its hair; it's so obviously a 'lady' doll that it's impossible to pretend it could be her baby. (For this reason she may appreciate such a doll in future years.)

One Christmas we saved up hard to buy Merle a huge brown bear, almost as tall as she was. We imagined it would be a real companion for her. I would never make that sort of mistake again. It proved to be much too overpowering for a comforting friend; it was just a big static object.

In the same way an animal which is too faithful a reproduction of an animal—you know, on all fours and without the big-eyed trimmings and floppy ears that make soft toys appealing—can't be treated as another small human. I remember when Brumas, the polar bear, was born at the Zoo, a costly but perfect toy version of her was brought out. Some people I know bought one for their three-year-old daughter, but she never played with it. She couldn't think of any games with a cast of one little girl and one polar bear . . .

There's the old joke, of course, of the father who buys his one-week-old son a train-set. Though I doubt if any father has actually done that, I've heard of one or two who've bought their *three*-year-olds train-sets, complete with electric points and reversing mechanisms and viaducts and heaven knows what else. Now if Father wants a train-set that badly for Christmas, I don't see why he shouldn't have one, and then his young son can play with *him* for as long as it interests the child. But don't let's pretend the train-set is a gift to anyone except Father. It's the same with the proper full-size football—ostensibly for the two-year-old. It's too big for the toddler and Father feels disappointed because he has to play all by himself.

Seriously, with the very best intentions one can waste an awful lot of money. The under-five is delightfully *un*materialistic; he doesn't appreciate something just because it cost a lot of money. A little girl of four-and-a-half once told me that her 'best' presents were her skipping-rope (20p) and her doll's pram (£12), in that order.

So the rocking-horse, the big bear, the dressed doll, the football, lie ignored in a corner, while your child plays with the approachable home-made stuffed elephant the old lady next door knitted for him.

And this is the moment to hide away some of the discarded toys. Most children get far more presents at Christmas than they can possibly cope with. They unwrap each parcel, look at it, handle it; but as the mountain grows, they don't really take in what the gift is. I've often seen my own children reach the stage where they're holding one thing in their hand while trying to open the next one. So when the present-opening is at last over and your child is absorbed in playing Battling Tops and showing off his new scooter, scoop up half of the barely-acknowledged gifts and put them away in a box upstairs.

Between Christmas and spring there are going to be an awful lot of days when the weather is bad and he can't play outside, when he's ill with a cold or perhaps even measles and needs cheering up, or when he's just plain fed up with everything he owns and wants a change. On any of those occasions you will be very glad that you have a box of 'new' toys upstairs with which to amuse him. Don't produce the boxful, though— that would only be repeating what you were trying to avoid at Christmas—but get out one or two things. And it's surprising, now that he has the time to study it, how fascinating Aunt Mary's puzzle will appear to him.

Before I leave the subject of Christmas, I ought to warn you about the well-meaning relative who gives your child a bag of sweets all to himself. A quarter-pound of chocolate in one go might please him very much, but on Christmas Day it is also likely to make him very sick. I cannot emphasise enough that children under five should not be given rich, exotic foods, nor sips from the wine-glasses of everybody in the room. Your *child* might tolerate the strange tastes very happily, but his digestive system won't. Nor, I suspect, will ours; but we're too old to learn.

HOLIDAYS

A 'date' which spreads over several dates is a summer holiday.

0 – 2 years

After much thought, I've come to the conclusion that on the whole I'm against taking a baby on holiday. We come back to the same old song: *babies like routine.* Unlike us, they do not long for a change of scene and the chance to meet new people. So the idea of an annual 'break' is meaningless to them. I admit the baby over a year might have fun playing on a sandy beach or bathing in a warm rockpool, with Mummy and Daddy nearby . . . assuming, of course, the weather is sunny and glorious. But in this country we cannot rely on the climate. And coping away from home in wet weather with a bored baby (because most of his playthings have had, for space reasons, to be left behind) is murder.

And I strongly advise you against taking your baby abroad. Even though you may find a travel firm who offer full board with accommodation in a little villa with a cooker on which to heat his food, and a private sink, bath and toilet—if the sunshine is all *that* guaranteed, then it's going to be too hot for Baby. Sunstroke, gastric troubles, disease can be sudden and serious in a baby.

And just think of all the stuff you'd have to take : bottles of Milton, packets of dried milk (the foreign milk may not be pasteurised), two dozen towelling nappies, a large Napisan and a bucket (and no promise of a launderette or a washing-machine at your destination), or a suitcase full of disposable nappies, and something like 15 lbs of tinned baby food for his dinners and teas!

In your own home he is surrounded by useful—by now, taken for granted—equipment. Leave his high-chair behind and you'll discover how difficult it is to feed a ten-month-old on your lap or on an ordinary dining chair. Leave his playpen, and you can't turn your back for two minutes. Leave his pram, and he'll have to walk or be carried everywhere. Leave his cot, and you'll have to hire one. And so on.

And this is true of holidays in Britain, too. Unless you drive a Rolls, or maybe a hardy van, you can't take everything and so you *automatically* suffer some inconvenience in going away. And returning to that sink and cooker . . . we spoiled twentieth-century beings have grown dependent on hot running water and laid-on cooking facilities in caring for our babies. For this reason I don't recommend camping or caravaning.

Now if you're about to argue that hotels have high-chairs, cots and so on, basins in the bedrooms and the cooking done for you, I agree; they do. But, boy, I think you'll regret it if you take your baby to a hotel. To start with, as I've stated earlier in this book, very few children under two are socially fit to eat with strangers. So if you have a thought for your fellow guests—and for your baby, who's doing his best, which is good enough for home, you'll feed him first. Then what happens to him while *you* eat? Or come to that, when you're in the lounge, or at the bar, or in the television room? To keep him sitting still or imprisoned in your bedroom is cruel and to allow him to crawl or march about is unfair to everybody else. And the nappies. Are you going to keep them in a pail beside the basin and wash them in the communal bathroom, or use disposables all the time and risk blocking up the plumbing? As a landlady myself I don't relish the thought of either alternative!

The answer is to stay at a hotel which caters specially for babies and young children, with meals planned specifically for them, nappy service, baby-sitting arrangements, trained nanny care, and all the trappings. But this sort of service will cost you plenty.

So will the other solution: hiring a holiday flat or cottage. You're on your own, with nobody to object to your baby playing in the middle of the floor, and you have all the facilities of home. But apart from gaining a change of air, are you really having a holiday, with all your usual chores to do but hampered by a peculiar vacuum-cleaner and an electric cooker when you're used to gas, or vice versa?

And for the money you'd pay out for a really good holiday cottage or a family-catering hotel for the three of you, you and your husband could have a package-deal holiday on the Continent or a luxurious one in this country.

And if you want or need a holiday so badly, then that is what I think the two of you should do: take it, but leave the baby behind with someone he loves. As I said in 'There is a Substitute for Mum': such a parting needs working up to gradually. Very few babies could accept more than a week in their first year, and not all even in their second. And if you have real doubts about whether your child will be happy with your sister Molly for two weeks, then don't go. You'd never relax for worrying about him! You'd do better to skip a holiday completely that year and put the saving towards a bumper family one when Junior is old enough to appreciate accompanying you.

2 – 5 years

And when is that? Not for several years yet I fear. The colour-picture in the brochures of mother, father and three children playing beach-cricket and the one showing them playing Monopoly in the comfortable custom-built holiday-chalet does not apply to us. Those children are never under five. There is no holiday activity which the family can all enjoy equally which would include a child of our age-group. Virtually everything you and your husband might want to do on your holiday conflicts with the needs and desires of your young child. You want to have a quiet drink at a shady table in an open-air café; your under five, once he's finished his bribe cold drink or ice-cream, wants to be off to play on the beach. You have been invited to a cocktail-party at the Palace Hotel by some rich acquaintances. However, the party will be between twelve and two, which, of course, is exactly when you give your three-year-old his lunch. He is engrossed in the Punch and Judy show but you want to drag him back to the hotel because it's drizzling. See what I mean?

You have spent fifty weeks of this year, never stopping for a cup of coffee when you are out shopping, turning down social invitations whenever you can't find a baby-sitter, going out for walks to feed the ducks when it's cold and you'd rather be indoors; and you painted a rosy picture for yourself of these two weeks being different. You imagined that your husband and child would play together, that he would enjoy building sand-castles, paddling, playing with a football and taking Junior for walks looking for pretty shells. And so he does—but only for about half an hour at a stretch. If you nag him to do more he's likely to resent you and the child and the money he has wasted on this holiday, and moan about having to 'work' during it. I know it's unfair, because he is a parent too; but that's the way it is. To add insult to injury, fathers are wont to complain when they see their wives washing children's clothes before being able to get out for the day and they grumble about the clobber of push-chair, sand-bucket and three cardigans which are vital issue for an hour on the beach.

Why only an hour when the sun's been shining all afternoon? Because your two-and-a-half-year-old sleeps from 2 o'clock till 3.30. I admit that most children over two can be trained out of sleep during the day, but one can't 'train' him out of getting tired and irritable. Once you've kept your child from his afternoon nap for fourteen days during your holiday, you'll find he won't go back to napping once he's home again. Bang goes that welcome break for you. It's a case of he'll still be tired but won't lie down.

These difficulties apart, an ordinary hotel, boarding-house or farm which accepts children but doesn't cater for them especially, is still no place for an under-five.

Moreover, the journey to your holiday-destination is something to be *endured* with a bored, fidgety, and possibly travel-sick child who wants to stop for potty every ten miles it seems.

All the objections are equally true of the holiday abroad, and I can add some more. 'The money your husband's wasting' is a larger amount for just the same old beach-routine; the trip to Venice you're missing because your child will be bored stiff and protesting, will hurt far more because you'll not see Italy again for quite some years to come; the leisurely swim with your husband in the warm waters of the Adriatic never happens because one of you has always to be in the shallows with the child.

G

Although not quite so menacing as with a baby, illness abroad is still a deterrent. Two to five-year-olds are more susceptible to infection than an older child; they are more likely to be affected by sunstroke. And if your child becomes ill while abroad, you either have to pay the doctor private fees or insure against medical expenses before you go. And don't forget communication with a doctor in a foreign language is going to be far from easy. Would you understand the doctor's instructions in Greek? Nursing a sick child in a hotel room or a villa under strange conditions and communicating your order for a lightly boiled egg and a glass of peach-juice in sign language to the chamber-maid could be a nightmare.

So what it amounts to is that you and your husband can have a holiday for yourselves or one for your child, but you can't have the two in one. Let's consider *your* holiday first. While you two fly off to Minorca, look at Viking Settlements in the Hebrides or take a dose of *Kultur* in Florence, it's back to that loving long-suffering Grandma with your child. If Grandmother in your family is unable to cope, it might be possible for you to make a reciprocal arrangement with close friends or neighbours. You mind their children for a fortnight in June, and come August they take over your Katie when you are in Florence or wherever.

Now we come to *your child's* holiday, which may be additional to your own or may have to be instead of it. The point is: you make up your minds beforehand that the holiday is mainly for the child's benefit, because the further he grows away from the age of two the more he will appreciate a new environment which is arranged for his benefit. So consider staying with friends who live in the country where there is a big garden, and possibly animals; where there is a meadow to play in and a shallow brook in which to paddle and throw sticks to float on the current.

Again you can rent a bungalow by the sea, or stay at a family-hotel. Another possibility with young children that might appeal to you is a holiday-camp. But be careful. Any advertisement offering 'child-minding facilities' may mean only that. I once visited the crèche in a holiday-camp. It was beautifully clean and full of lovely toys of the rocking-horse/big doll variety. It would have driven any Playgroup Leader to drink. There was nothing for the children to play with in a creative sense and the fifteen or eighteen children I saw there were either apathetic or grizzling. The young nurses in attendance seemed medically competent and kind, *but*...

Don't submit yourselves to come home from your annual holiday with 'buts'. Be honest about what you hope to get out of your holiday and then go after that. Bon Voyage!

CHAPTER TWELVE

How do I Tell my Child About...?

CHILDREN ASK questions endlessly; and children between two and five especially, who are too young to be taught at school or to learn through reading, badger their parents with 'why's', because asking is a way of finding out. I'm not talking about the 'why' game—whatever reply Mother or Father gives, the child says: 'Why?' It goes on and on until the exasperated, exhausted parent shouts: 'Because I say so!' That child doesn't even listen to the answers; he's merely clutching at attention. No, I'm speaking of the very genuine questions that young children put to their parents, and what we, as adults, should tell them. In a word, I would say the truth. I consider that all questions should be answered honestly and attentively.

'Why can't we go to the shops, Mummy?'

'Because the people who work there have gone home, and the shops are closed.'

'Why do we eat dinner?'

'Because eating helps us to grow and keep strong.'

'Why is it dark at night time?'

'Because we no longer face the sun.'

'Is it night-time everywhere?'

'Well, no . . .' It's amazing what we as adults learn in answering our children correctly!

As a general rule, I would recommend you answer only what is asked, because that's as much as he can understand. If he is capable of taking in more or if your reply doesn't satisfy him, he will ask the rider: like 'Is it night-time everywhere?' If he still seems interested and you are tempted to elaborate, without prompt from him—well, it's a communication between you and that never did anyone any harm. But don't kid yourself you're teaching him anything further. You're not. It is only an older child who can grasp the extensions of a subject he's never even wondered about before. Of course, if your under-five looks puzzled by your reply, that's as good as saying : 'Hey, I don't get you; come again . . .' And in that case by all means try re-phrasing your answer, but still only that one answer.

And may I warn you that some things you will be asked over and over again. This isn't due to forgetfulness on your child's part, but rather because the answer takes time to be absorbed. Stars aren't little lights; they're different suns. Strange, that. Babies come from their mothers' tummies. Even more improbable—*he* came out of yours !

Mentioning pregnancy and birth leads me to say that there have always been 'awkward' questions which young children ask, one of them being about sex. I'd like to deal with the per-sistent ones in detail, so that you will be prepared if the topic comes up in your household. So let's start with How Do I Tell My Child about . . . Sex?

SEX

Let me say at the outset that, regrettably, children to not wait till a cosy autumn evening round the fire to ask 'Mummy, where did I come from ?' The topic is just as likely to arise in the bus-queue, where confounded onlookers are bound to titter. But wherever your child asks the question, your answer should be the same : from my tummy. Naturally, this is far easier for him to comprehend if you are pregnant. He sees your tummy grow-ing; towards the end of the nine months, he may even be able to feel the baby's movements. But even if you yourself are not pregnant when he is between three and five, it is probably that a close friend of yours will be. So you can talk about the baby in her tummy instead.

And contrary to what some people might believe : the fact that babies grow in their mummies' tummies may be all your child wants to know about the subject for the whole age-span of our book. If so, let him be. He'll get around to it again sometime in the future. (And it is just possible even that much won't interest him.) But it is more probable that he'll want to know how the baby got in there, in which case you say Daddy planted a seed, and the baby grew from that. You can illustrate this with the bulbs and seeds you plant in the garden, which grow into much bigger flowers. Another aspect that often worries children is how the baby is going to get out. To this, I've said 'through a little tunnel between his mother's legs'. All right, you argue, they're the easy ones; how about the 64,000 dollar one: *how* did Daddy plant this seed? Frankly, I've yet to meet a four-year-old who *volunteered* this question. But if yours does, then answer: 'With his penis'. If the truth is too absurd, too shattering for him to accept as yet, then he'll simply forget about it until he is ready. Don't be afraid that telling him about the sexual function of a penis is going to plague his mind with thoughts of Sin and Shame. This would happen only if your attitude when you spoke of sex was ashamed or salacious; providing you remain matter of fact, so will your child. It is too early in his life to connect the making of babies with an expression of deep emotion.

If you are surprised or shocked that I should suggest using the name 'penis' to a young child, I make no apology. I abhor twee names for the sexual organs; more, I believe that automatically using the real ones eases discussion and attitude about sex later on in early adolescence and even beyond in actual love-making. So I would suggest you teach your child the words 'penis', 'vagina', 'breast', 'testicles' as he or she needs such vocabulary.

This brings me to another tricky point. How does a little girl without a brother learn what a penis is? As I said earlier, I very much doubt if she'll care yet how that seed got inside; but if she does, there's always the hope that she'll have watched some baby boy relation or neighbour being bathed.

Or perhaps her daddy is one of the people who don't mind the family wandering in and out when he's sitting in the bath. If so, the problem is solved. But I am not for one moment suggesting you and your husband adopt standards which you consider immodest, for the sake of your children's sex education. In the last decade or so, some experts have advocated nudity in the home because they believed it would prevent the next generation growing up inhibited. And I'm sure it has, where parents treated it as a matter of course that their children would from time to time see them naked. But in families where the parents felt embarrassed about stripping off but nevertheless heroically did so, it has often had the reverse effect. The embarrassment transmitted itself to the children and they have grown up more inhibited than ever. Conversely, too much flaunting liberalism over nudity can disturb a child. So I would say : stick to your own standards. If the worst comes to the worst, the brotherless little girl can always be told that a penis is rather like a finger, can't she ?

What about the birds and the bees for sex education ? Well, the reproduction of birds and bees specifically is far too theoretical for an under-five, and it does presuppose that you are well-informed about the sex-life of the bee . . . But actually watching the birth of your bitch's pups or the guinea-pig across the road having her babies—that's excellent for your child, an experience he will treasure. Country children who have watched the lambings, etc., perhaps even the mating too, ever since they can remember, almost always grow up with a healthy, natural attitude towards birth and sexual organs. They, of course, will have watched hundreds of young animals being suckled by their mothers. And this is something that any town child can see as well—a cat nursing her kittens, a mare in a field giving milk to her foal, a monkey at the zoo with her new-born baby. Take every opportunity of pointing this out to your child, and explain that this is the way the mother feeds her baby : from her own body. It is even better, of course, if your child can watch you breast-feeding his younger brother or sister. Or perhaps you have a friend who *honestly* wouldn't mind him watching her nurse. The more he can learn about sex as he learns about everything else, the better.

TALKING TO STRANGERS

If you abide by my rule of not letting your child wander about on his own, the number of chances of his talking to the wrong sort of stranger is limited, isn't it ? Even so, I know that there are occasions when one parent out of a group goes down to the park playground or along to the nursery school to escort all the children home; and this would be an opportunity on which a stranger could step in and pose as 'the person Mummy sent'. How do you guard against such a thing? Firstly, you promise your child that you will never ever send someone he doesn't know as your ambassador, and secondly you instil into him from the very first time he plays outside that he must not under any circumstances speak to strangers or take sweets from them. (You needn't frighten him with reasons; the under-five has to take an awful lot of rules on your say-so.) To underline this point, I even handed back chocolates elderly ladies kindly offered my own children in the park. 'I'm afraid they're not allowed to accept sweets from strangers,' I explained. 'But thank you all the same.'

THE FACT HE'S ADOPTED

I don't think you can better the well-tried method of a story of how you came to choose him. It should be among the first stories you tell your child and it will become such a favourite you will probably have to repeat it time and time again. 'Once upon a time Mummy and Daddy were very lonely because they had no little boy or girl to live with them. So they went to a big white stone house where there were a lot of children who had no mothers and fathers.' Elaborate it; take it slowly. Tell how 'the nurse in charge took you along a room, and in the fourth cot was a lovely little boy, and he was wearing blue rompers. And he smiled at you, and you both smiled back. And then you played peepbo together, and you loved each other very much. And then you were allowed to take him home. And that little boy was YOU.' As he grows older, you can go into even more details about your journey home, and how he first saw his own room, and what Teddy thought of him when they said 'hello', etc., etc.

But don't fall into the trap of suggesting you chose him because he was pretty, or because you wanted a brother for your own daughter, or because he was a new baby . . . You chose him BECAUSE HE WAS HIMSELF. And however it may have started out, now you do love him for himself, don't you?

Later on, of course, he is going to ask what happened to his real Mummy. Don't be hurt by this question; he asks it because he is curious, not because he loves you less. He deserves an honest answer—as honest as is possible without wounding him. 'She died. Or she hadn't a Daddy to help her look after you, and so she asked the nurse in the big white house to find you a Mummy and Daddy, and we loved you so much she picked us.' It's strange, but although children adopted as babies can't remember their natural parents and therefore can have no love for them, the biological link, particularly with the mother, is so strong that to learn they were *deserted* can have serious psychological repercussions. That's why an adopted child can usually accept that his real mother died (because she had no choice about leaving him), but not that she abandoned him in a church porch.

While speaking of the adopted child, may I put in a plea not to over-compensate him for the deprivation of his natural parents? You are already giving him what he needs most in the world : the deep love you would give a son or daughter you had conceived yourselves. So once you have adopted a child, treat him as your own. Smack him when he's spiteful; deny him sweets that would harm his teeth; refuse to sit by his cot all evening. In other words, let him grow up into a reasonable human being.

REMARRIAGES

Introducing a stepmother or stepfather into the home is never simple, admittedly; but I don't believe it is quite as difficult as the romantic novels would have us believe. Their idea of Father going away to Spain for the summer and returning with a beautiful bride whom the children have never seen doesn't happen in real life—or at least I hope it doesn't. In practice, surely, the children already know Helen. She's a friend who comes to tea on Sundays, who helps bath them before she and Daddy go out for the evening, who cooked for them at Christmas. If this isn't the case, then I think it ought to be, before the day that Daddy tells his children that Helen is coming to live with them permanently. Or, in the case of a stepfather, he has played ball with them in the garden; he has come on holiday to the seaside with them; he has answered their questions.

The point I'm making is that Helen or Joe are friends of the children, quite apart from their relationship with the parent. And that is how I think they should approach their new role after the wedding-day as well : as a *friend*, not as a substitute Mummy or Daddy. I believe that much of the resentment over stepmothers and fathers can be put down to the children's feeling that they are usurping a position held by someone very dear to them. It might even be better if the children called them 'Helen' or 'Joe' rather than 'Mummy' or 'Daddy'. In fact I know of a delightful instance where the stepmother was called by her Christian name to start with, but after a year or so she became 'Mummy' instead. Nobody suggested the change; it wasn't even a conscious one. She had simply grown into her new title.

Equally to potential step-parents, I would say : don't expect to love your fiancé's children as you would your own. Like them, as people in their own right and not only as an adjunct of your beloved. And once you are married, don't be so anxious to please the children, you allow yourself to be an over-indulgent and bad parent. A step-parent must assume all the responsibilities of parenthood—protection, correction and attention. Remember, we are talking in this book of children under five.

If you really cannot abide your fiancé's child or, as happens more often, your child hates your intended (probably due to jealousy), I would strongly advise you to postpone your wedding plans until the relationship improves. Let the potential step-parent and the child spend time alone together; for instance, a game of football for 'the men' might just do the trick. And if at the end of say a year, the situation is no better, than I would seriously re-consider whether this marriage is right for you. Taking sides in a war between your husband and your child—or being the cause of one between your new wife and her jealous little son—will tear you apart.

DEATH

What you tell your child happens to people when they die will largely depend on your own religious beliefs. If you believe your late mother has gone 'to heaven', then that is what you say. A three or four-year-old will be satisfied to learn Grandma has gone to a peaceful other world. If you don't accept any form of life-after-death, then I would suggest you describe Grandma as having gone to sleep for ever. Your child will have seen people asleep—old people in their chairs, babies in their prams, perhaps even Daddy on a Sunday morning—and know it's a quiet, relaxed state to be in. At any event, I think children should be told when a member of their family has died. Death is a sad subject, but it's one we all have to learn to accept.

If there is a dead bird on the lawn, don't pretend it's invisible. You should tell your child calmly and sympathetically that the bird has died because there's been a week of snow and no food for it. And later you discreetly dispose of the corpse. If your dog kills a rabbit, explain to your child that dogs, left wild and living without a family who feeds them dog-food, eat rabbits to live. Cats kill birds, but in turn birds eat worms. Young children are not so appalled by the cruelty of nature as one might think. Sometimes, though, they do go through a morbid phase, when for weeks on end they keep asking you about death. If your child reacts in this way, don't be alarmed; it's one of those subjects that takes a lot of absorbing.

Finally, I would say that it is a mistake to let your child see the body of someone dear to him who has died. The decomposition in only a day or two is unflattering, and to a child grotesque and unpleasant. It is far better for him to remember that person as he or she was.

I would even extend that to cover very ill people. Such a sick-bed would be a frightening place to a young child. By all means, let him send messages, even better a painting or gift he has made; but don't inflict visits upon him.

COLOUR

I include this because an innocent question like 'Why has that lady got a black skin . . . or a white skin, or a yellow skin or any other shade of skin?' has apparently become an emotive one. I've heard of a mother who was asked just this question by her three-year-old and didn't know how to answer it without being racial.

Isn't the easiest, most frank answer the basic geographical

one? That she has a black skin because she (or her mother and father) comes from a hot country where the sun always shines and the people are dark, to protect them from it. Or she has a white skin because she comes from England where the sun never seems to shine and the people never get a chance even to get suntanned, etc. etc.

SEPARATION OR DIVORCE

There is no painless way of telling a child that his mother or father will not be living with him any more. But at least you can stop the knife going in even deeper by saying that 'Daddy has *left* us'. As we said when talking about adoption, children cannot bear to have been *deserted* by their parents, abandoned because they didn't care. So however bitter you may feel about the break-up of your marriage, try to reassure your child that Daddy still loves him. He has gone away only because he couldn't be happy living in this house with you both. (Say this even if it isn't the whole truth, in order to persuade him his father loves him.) And wherever possible, permit your child to continue to have some sort of relationship with his absented parent.

CHAPTER THIRTEEN

A Spoonful of Sugar Helps . . .

According to Mary Poppins, a spoonful of sugar helps the medicine go down when looking after a sick child. *Our* spoonful of sugar comes in extra glucose for energy, extra loving attention for comfort, and the sweetness of rediscovering one's well-beloved old toys.

How do you know when your child is not well? When a normally happy and active child becomes listless and fretful and loses interest in his surroundings—this is often the first sign that he's 'sickening for something'. Since a baby or toddler can't tell you where it hurts, you have to make a few investigations. First take his temperature. Put him on your lap and soothe him until he's somewhat comforted. It is difficult to keep the thermometer in place while your child is struggling and protesting. Do not take his temperature anywhere *except in the groin*. The mercury bulb has to lie next to the skin in the fold between his body and his thigh, and be kept there for two full minutes by your watch. I've found the easiest way to do this is by crossing his knees and pressing your hand firmly against the thigh. If his temperature is slightly above 99°F. (37°C.), then he is probably only going in for a cold. If it's above 101°, inform your doctor immediately. Also watch out for the opposite, which is that the thermometer reading is 95°F. or below, and the child's skin feels cold and clammy. The doctor should be told about this one too.

In addition, check for rashes; and whether his nose is so blocked he'd have trouble eating and drinking, or whether he has the typical barking cough of croup. Vomiting and diarrhoea together, particularly in a small baby, are danger signals requiring very urgent medical attention. Ear-discharge and ear-ache, undue coughing or tummy-ache are other indications that something is seriously amiss. I hardly need to mention that a child who has fits or convulsions, or who has swallowed something like a hairclip, pin or the red iron pills you didn't lock up safely, needs a doctor at once.

It is wrong to try to diagnose your child's illness and to treat him yourself without medical advice. The important thing is to let your doctor know what the symptoms are and *let him decide* whether he needs to visit. He may instruct you over the telephone, which is fine; but carry out those instructions conscientiously and ring back when asked to or if your small patient's condition gets worse. It's never a good thing to cart your baby or toddler to a crowded waiting room, especially when he's ill. That's why I consider that the doctor should come to your home, if he needs to see the child.

Ideally you should call your doctor during surgery hours, but certainly in the daytime. It is very rare that a child's illness, except if it is a sudden emergency, starts after midnight. Many doctors complain about the night calls they have to children who have been ill since before lunch. So contact your doctor when you first *think* you may need his help—not at 2 o'clock in the morning when you jolly well *know* you do.

If you don't have a telephone in the house, do not leave your child alone while you dash up to the call-box. Ask a neighbour to phone for you, and if all your neighbours are out, stop a passer-by. Very few people will refuse to summon a doctor to a sick child.

If you have left a message at the doctor's surgery and he hasn't called within six hours or less and your child seems worse, dial 999 and ask for an ambulance, and go with him to the hospital.

When your doctor does call, have a clean towel waiting for him in the bathroom and a good light available in the sick-room. In cold weather make sure that the child's bedroom is warm all the time, but particularly during the doctor's visit because he's going to be exposed during an examination. If your child sleeps in a bunk bed with a brother or sister, do bear in mind your doctor can't get at him in there—either top level or bottom. So clear the living-room of the rest of the family and lay him on the settee for the doctor's visit. Incidentally, do stick around : your presence will give your child comfort and confidence, and besides, it is you, not the three-year-old, who has to prepare a light diet and give lots of fluids or whatever?

Never give a child medicines prescribed or bought for someone else, or even the remainder of those prescribed for him on a previous occasion. Part of the purpose of the doctor's visit is to prescribe the right medicine for this particular illness. And once you have a prescription, get it to a chemist as soon as possible— not ten hours later when your husband comes home. So once again you're going to have to utilise a neighbour, or even a stranger if treatment is required that urgently.

Now tempting though it may sound, double the dose in half the time won't make your child better twice as fast. It could even make him a great deal more sick. So carry out the precise dosage instructions. And don't stop the treatment just because your child seems a bit better. If the doctor said he needed a full bottle of red medicine, then that's what he needs . . . even if it takes him a further four days after he's fit to finish it up.

Apart from any specific instructions the doctor gives, I would advise that any child with a temperature of over 100°F. should be kept in bed. The toilet is usually a cold place in winter so a pot in his room is a Must. If your child is still in nappies, you should change him in his cot. The process of being washed may make a sick child tetchy but that's no reason for not maintaining hygiene. In illnesses accompanied by fever it is even more important to keep him clean and his *teeth brushed*.

If a child is seriously ill and is being nursed at home, a daily blanket-bath is beneficial. Now this needs a little forethought. First the warm room again. Next you'll need a bowl of warm water, with Infacare in the water (even if he has graduated to soap ordinarily), his own flannel or sponge, a warmed towel and clean warmed pyjamas ready. Cover the bed or cot with a waterproof sheet, then cover this with a spare blanket and put the child on top; cover the child with a second spare blanket. (Spare blankets must be well aired and warmed!) Now take off his pyjamas under his bathblanket and wash a small part of his body, and dry. Only expose the part you are washing, not the whole child. When you have finished, whip out the bathblankets and waterproof cover, dress the child in clean night-things and tuck him up again. For cleaning teeth use a pail for spitting into and a tooth-mug and usual brush and paste.

I think it's worth mentioning that for colds or other respiratory infections it helps to drain the air-passages if you tip the cot or bed at the foot-end. A pair of ordinary bricks placed lengthways, one under each leg, serve admirably. This means that the child's feet are about four inches higher than his head. Pad the head-end of the cot!

Now I know from experience and I'm sure you do too, that when one is ill one gets heartily sick of lying in one's bed and looking at the bedroom walls for days on end. For this reason I suggest that your sick child is nursed on a bed made up with sheets and blankets in the living-room on the settee and goes to his own bedroom at his usual bed-time. The room can be aired in the meantime and his own bed will be fresh and much nicer to spend the night in. Apart from its being a change to come downstairs, he has the advantage of your company; he can watch all the other activities that go on downstairs and the television is there.

Unlike an adult patient, children don't knit, read or do cross-word puzzles, but they do need to play and have things to do. It would be rare that a child who is allowed to be nursed at home is so ill that he hasn't the energy to sit up and play in his sickbed. First of all his usual bed-companions will be welcome and oddly enough he will often prefer an old much-used, no longer smart rabbit to the new birthday doll. And no adult chooses the moment when he has a raging temperature to conquer Sartre—so with a child. He does not want the challenge of games which stretch him; he wants a puzzle he can solve, a castle he can build, a picture-book he knows by heart. So fish out the toys you thought he'd outgrown a year ago and they'll make a triumphant come-back. Many games need a flat hard surface, so he'll probably need a tray. An even better piece of equipment is a cantilever-table (often offered cheaply by mail-order houses). I've got one myself, and apart from finding it mighty useful when nursing my family, it makes a luxurious bedside-table for guests or a super breakfast-table for a spoiled husband.

Take convalescence gently. Your child should not be up until his temperature is right down and then only for half a day at first. Dress him promptly when he first gets up again— the floor is draughty! Don't take him out for a walk until he has been up for a normal day, and watch the weather. Over-dressing a child in warm weather is as detrimental as letting him catch cold in the winter weather.

Before I leave this chapter may I remind you of something I said in 'To Love Honour and Obey'. In the name of good discipline you must gradually withdraw any special indulgences of sickness during convalescence—otherwise they'll become bad habits!

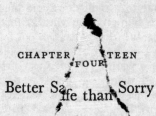

CHAPTER FOURTEEN

Better Safe than Sorry

THE ROYAL Society for the Prevention of Accidents has helped me prepare this chapter for you on how to avoid mishaps—mishaps which are all too often fatal. Of the black annual total of 8,000 deaths in the home, three-quarters are elderly people and *children under five*. That figure is even more horrific when you consider that in most cases a little forethought would have saved them. The same applies to children killed on the roads —900 of them every year. I'm ashamed to add that at least 150 of these are infants in our age-group who are out in the streets unaccompanied.

Harassed mothers say, 'Oh, if you must have an ice-cream, here's the money; go and buy one,' hardly considering that the sweetshop is on a main road . . . Or they leave their two-year-old in the care of his older brother, and the older brother, hardly surprisingly, gets bored with Tommy tagging along and sort of forgets about him. Or perhaps the milkman leaves the back door open, and Tommy simply wanders out. Not the mother's fault then, not really the milkman's fault. But if Tommy is hit by a car, *he may still be killed regardless.*

While your children are small, you must be on constant alert. If the house has been suspiciously peaceful for the last ten minutes, jump to it; find out why. To a toddler, Mummy's vaguely-remembered warning about not stepping off the kerb doesn't get a look in when his ball's rolled in that direction. In two cases out of three, he'll dash after it.

Remember that from eighteen months to four, he is full of adventure and curiosity, but his understanding is less developed. He has hardly any sense of prudence, and his attention span is limited. He is intelligent enough to know how to stand on a chair and reach up to things, but doesn't understand enough yet to foresee the results of his so doing. He will be able to open the garden gate, but will not realise the dangers beyond.

I'm deliberately painting a frightening picture because the penalties for carelessness are so severe. Even when the accident doesn't cost your child his life, it causes him suffering; it could maim him physically or emotionally; and it will certainly add to the burden carried by our Health Service. So I ask you to read this chapter carefully, absorb its warnings, and then get on with the business of teaching your child to live. I'd be the last person to recommend you sit there considering every crisis that could occur in any given contingency. For instance, arguing that if you let your fifteen-month-old push his dog-on-wheels about, it might run away with him, and he could fall down and hit his chin on the hearth, and that could knock out his teeth. Sure, all those things might happen—*might*—but he's got to live, not merely exist. Only by wrapping him in cotton-wool can you protect him from every danger, and as we've said earlier in this book, that philosophy brings its own problems.

The point is : don't ask for trouble. And as your child's comprehension increases, explain to him *why* he mustn't do certain things. Eventually you'll be rewarded by his telling you—about the matches or an oncoming car, etc. To start with, of course, you won't be able to reason with him at all. So let's begin with Safety First for a baby.

And as we go along, I've asked the Red Cross to explain what you do if, despite precautions, your child does meet with an accident. Needless to say, the treatment they prescribe holds good for any age patient—seven days to seventy years.

– *1 year*

You can prevent some accidents before he's even born. Check that the equipment you buy him—his cot, his playpen, his baby-chair, etc.—all carry the 'Kite Mark', showing they are made to BSI safety requirements. This will assure that his head can't jam between bars or his high-chair collapse when he leans back. And take added care when selecting his pram. By all means fall in love with an acid-yellow one, but before signing the cheque, do make sure the design is safe for you as well as noticing the colour.

Walk round the shop a bit it; see how the handle feels. If it's an uncomfortable height with you, you run the risk of leaning on it too heavily and thereby tipping the pram over. The same thing happens to mothers who persist in hanging shopping-bags over the handle, or even slinging a bag over an arm that holds the pram: it upsets the balance. The proper place for shopping is on a tray underneath the chassis.

If you're a half-pint, check that you can see over the hood when it's up. After all, you can't drive properly with a curtain over the windscreen! And pay special attention to the brake. Would you trust it on an incline in wet, slippery weather? If the answer's no, frankly I think I'd find another pram. A good brake is imperative, and you should use it even when you've only stopped to fish out your mac hat.

In the pram's instruction manual about regular servicing and professional repairs, the manufacturers remind you of the importance of assembling your pram correctly, referring to the kind where you can detach the wheels for storage and travelling. There are screws which have to be tightened and rings which have to be slid over certain bits. Take a tip from a young mother I know who dare not take her pram apart: don't trust the assistant's word that the chassis comes off in a trice have a go yourself—yes, there in the shop, with an impatient queue of customers behind you. Make sure that you can do it, and in a reasonable time. It isn't much good your husband' being able to bash that chassis into its rest, if he's going to be away at work when you need to get the two halves in and out of the car. And to use the pram incorrectly assembled wobbling somewhere around the middle, could have hideous consequences.

Finally check that the pram has sensible anchor points for a harness. I've seen poor babies pinned like butterflies on board because their harness rings were in the wrong position

And having got the rings for a harness, buy him the harness. (Leather ones look grand, but generally speaking plain ordinary webbing proves more comfortable.) That pram's a long way up; your baby really does need to be strapped in to stop him falling, or clambering, out. Slipping one side undone 'to give him more freedom' is almost worse than no harness at all : because if he did fall under those circumstances, he'd be left hanging. Actually, there's a case for using a harness immediately he attempts to haul himself up, just in case the first occasion on which he succeeds he's alone in his pram.

Another sensible safety measure is to buy a net for it. They protect him against cats, birds, toddlers' curious fingers; and when travelling in the car in the chassis-part or in a carry-cot, they're an added 'holder-inner'. Incidentally, always *wedge* a carry-cot on to the back seat of a car, so that it can't slide off or tip up if the driver should have to stop suddenly. A carry-cot restraining device is now obtainable from the K. L. Jeenay range of goods.

Until a child walks, obviously there can be no question of road drill. Nevertheless, I would draw *your* attention to the danger of pushing a pram out into the road from between parked vehicles or by a bend, and then peering out yourself to see if the coast is clear. Or, rather, *was* clear. If there had been a car coming, the pram would have already been hit ! And another thing : before you had the baby, you may have been awfully nippy about dodging through moving traffic. With a pram, that's much too difficult. It's a big long thing, and it isn't pliable—*and your precious baby is inside it*. I know it's a bore, but make the effort to walk along to a pedestrian crossing. Why, drivers have even been known to smile as they wave virtuous mothers across the zebra...

In our chapters on feeding and hygiene, we have already discussed the need for sterilisation to kill germs. But infection isn't the only danger connected with feeding. Of all fatal accidents in the home, by far the greatest killer among *babies* is

KING. The majority of these are victims of a propped-up bottle (see page 19, but some merely bring back a feed when they're in their cot and, because they cannot yet turn away, they inhale the vomit and choke, which prevents them from breathing. Frightening thought. But the risk is almost nullified if you always lay baby on his side or stomach . . . not on his back.

If your baby is choking, the first thing to do is to hook out with your finger the particle of food or scrap of material, etc., which is obstructing his throat. Then hold him upside down by his ankles with one hand, and give several firm thumps between his shoulders with the other.

Another point about feeding: you can bet your life that if you ever forget to carry out the wrist-test on his milk, that'll be the occasion when it will be too hot and SCALD his mouth. Solution: don't forget. Always check that a liquid is at most at blood temperature before your baby tells you it isn't!

The other hackneyed test is the elbow one for bath-water. Well, before you decide that's far too tepid a temperature and pour in an extra couple of gallons of hot (always, incidentally, put the cold water in first), just test your own bath-water the same way. You'll begin to agree that your hands are considerably tougher than the rest of your body.

However, even in the best regulated homes, young children do suffer scalds and here's what to do about it. Forget the outdated butter routine, and for that matter any other creams. Plain cool water's the thing. The aim is to reduce the skin temperature, and the fastest way of doing that is to immerse the damaged area in cold water—not so icy he suffers shock, of course. By all means chuck the contents of the water-jug over him if that's within grabbing distance, but ideally you need a *continuous* flooding.

Therefore I'd suggest you THINK SINK—it's a convenient bath for a scalded under-five, and you can keep the burnt arms or whatever in it until the pain has subsided, which can be anything from minutes upwards, according to how severe the injury is.

Remove any steaming clothes. (If you've ever plunged a rubber-gloved hand into the washing-machine only to find there's a hole in one finger, you'll know how that glove retains the heat!) When the worst of the burn, and a scald is a wet burn, has gone, pat him dry and cover the injured area with a clean dry bandage loosely. And if that area is larger than the size of his hand, it's serious; your child should be seen by a doctor.

Also on the subject of hot water: use a large sponge for bathing. Babies sometimes put small soft ones into their mouths and choke.

Another treacherous plaything, surprisingly, is his talc. Inhaled powder can obstruct the air passages. Now, if your baby's anything like mine were he'll want to hold the talcum-powder every time you use it on him. I don't see any harm in this, providing you check that it's done up when he takes it. (Worth doing anyway to save your carpet and clothes being covered in white dust!) The important thing is not to leave him playing with the talc afterwards in his cot. He could get it undone, and then the danger could start.

Need I ever say: never leave him alone in the bath for a second? He can drown in a very few inches of water and fearfully quickly owing to the fact that at this age he won't put up any struggle. This seems a good moment to tell you about The Kiss of Life: the treatment for ASPHYXIA.

This is a dramatic name for MOUTH-TO-MOUTH ARTIFICIAL RESPIRATION, and you should employ it at once whenever breathing has stopped. I know babies breathe so quietly that many a mother has woken up her first-born just to check he's still alive! But that's usually in the dark. In daylight she should be able to see his chest moving up and down. So if you can't see any such movement and you can't hear your baby exhaling either, check his breath against a mirror; it should steam up. If it doesn't, quick—start the mouth-to-mouth resuscitation. I hardly need add that if you rescue his limp, silent form from under water, you don't delay hunting through three old handbags for a mirror to assure yourself that he isn't breathing. If he's not coughing, he's not breathing either under those circumstances.

Now place him on his back, and with one hand press his forehead down and with the other lift his chin up. This prevents his tongue from obstructing the back of his throat. Maintain this position all the time.

1. Take a deep breath.

2. Open your mouth. Seal your lips round your baby's
mouth and nose.

3. Puff air very gently but firmly into his mouth and so
into his lungs.

4. Remove your mouth, turning your head to look at his
chest, which should have risen and now be falling as the
air comes out.

Repeat the cycle 1–4.

Continue puffing at a steady rate until he can breathe for
himself. At that stage, turn him on his side because he may
vomit.

If on the other hand, his skin remains blue-grey in colour,
the carotid pulse at the side of the neck is absent, and his
pupils are widely dilated, then his heart has ceased beating,
too. Keep calm; there's something you can do about that as
well. Officially it's called EXTERNAL HEART COMPRESSION.

First of all slap his chest smartly over the lower part of the
breastbone. That in itself is often enough to start the beat. If it
fails, overcome your desperation and put two fingers on the
lower half of the breastbone, keeping your palm off his chest.
Then press the breastbone down firmly with a rocking movement fifteen times, which should take about nine seconds. Then
quickly and smoothly alternate with two more inflations of the
lung. (To live, a person needs to breathe and his heart has to
beat.) Eventually you should be rewarded by both a flickery
pulse and a few gasps.

If you've been trying unsuccessfully for say fifteen minutes,
break off and dial 999 for an ambulance. But don't do that
precipitately because the half-minute it'll take you to get
through could be fatal for your baby. Obviously, if there's
someone else available, get him or her to phone at once while
you get on with the treatment, and afterwards that other person can do the heart-massage while you look after the breathing. But it should still be an *alternate* treatment—heart-lung,
heart-lung—but *two* people can make it more effective by giving *one* inflation of the lung to five presses on the breastbone.

Now it is just possible that in a very cold atmosphere a new
baby can stop breathing. He hasn't suffocated or drowned or

swallowed anything; his only symptom is that he is deathly cold to the touch. This is HYPOTHERMIA—loss of body heat.

Whenever a person stops breathing, that is your first priority : mouth-to-mouth resuscitation. Once breathing is re-established, you should gradually raise your baby's body temperature by wrapping him in blankets and giving him warm milk to drink, providing, of course, he is conscious. Do not toss him about 'to get the circulation going'—his little body needs all the energy it's got simply to survive.

Since mothers have become aware of the danger of hypothermia, however, there have been far more two-month-olds panting under three woollies in a heatwave than fading away in some cold dark castle. Still, it's something to bear in mind, especially for a winter babe. Ideally his room temperature shouldn't fall below 65°, which means that on a snowy night he's going to need all-night heating in there. Not a naked flame, please. Preferably a small convector or the central heating left on in his room only. Never, never leave him alone with an oil-stove. Personally, with young children in the house, I would re-examine alternatives to heating with an oil-stove, altogether.

But however cold the weather may be, don't be tempted to leave a hot-water bottle or electric pad in your baby's cot with him. It's just asking for burns and scalds. Pop them in while he's out being fed, and take them out when you put him back, if you follow me. Besides, if he's wearing a stretch sleeping-suit (and I approve of them whole-heartedly) he won't be quite so susceptible to cold sheets on bare legs, the way we are !

Another advantage of those suits is that they have no nasty little ribbons round the neck. Apart from the fact your ingenious baby will drive you mad by pulling them out, he just might get one half-out, roll over awkwardly and strangle himself with it.

And while we're on the subject : beware his glorious christening shawl. His fingers could become entangled in those lacy patterns and serious harm could result.

Ah yes, and although there are pretty pillow-slips in the shops with 'baby' embroidered in one corner, pillows for babies are both unnecessary and dangerous—due to the risk of suffo-

cation. When your baby is old enough to sit up in his pram,
he can have a pillow tucked behind his back for comfort. But
it should be taken away whenever he lies down. If you can
avoid using a pillow in his cot or bed until he is old enough
to ask for one, all the better. My own children didn't ask for
pillows until they were old enough to want to sit up in bed
to read before getting-up time. The spine and back muscles
grow more strong for being allowed to function correctly.

Finally, for this age-group and the next, make sure his
toys (or anything else you give him to play with, like a spoon)
are small enough for him to hold safely, but too large to
swallow. And remember that plastic breaks easily; so be on the
look-out for bits that snap off.

1 – 2 years

Safety-wise, this is a nightmare era. Your baby is fully mobile,
but none too steady with it, and he wants to touch everything
he sees. BURNS are the worst enemy here. So let's kick off with
some big dos and don'ts.

1. Use a fixed fireguard round all fires, and designate
   the fireplace a prohibited area, even when it's not
   alight.
2. Keep matches right away from your child. Their boxes
   are small and rattly, and have instant-infant appeal.
   You have been warned.
3. Never air nappies, or anything else, on the fireguard.
   Flapping there, they're more than likely to catch
   alight.
4. Buy flame-resistant clothes and fabrics for nightwear.
   They can save those all-too-common sleepy winter
   casualties.

If ever your toddler does burn himself, first put out any flames
by rolling him in a blanket or coat; and then tear off smoulder-
ing clothes by seizing them in a part where they're not burning.
(Otherwise there'll be two of you in hospital!) Never prick
blisters or slap on soap. Simply follow the cool-water treatment
I've described for scalds. And if you're only seconds away

from water, it's better not to remove clothes—because anything burnt is sterile.

If you need to call an ambulance (because there is bleeding or the burn area is large) work in this order :

1. Close doors and windows on the fire to contain it, and move small fellow to somewhere safe.
2. Treat him for burns.
3. Leave him on the floor with a clean damp cloth over the burn while you ring for an ambulance.
4. Put out the fire. Remember you can always buy a new home; you can never buy a new baby.

Though less of a killer statistically, there are more cases of scalding than burning in this age-group. It stands to reason; we know fire is a potential menace but we tend to treat hot, even boiling, water as a household amenity. We forget its danger to crawlers and toddlers. RoSPA (Royal Society for the Prevention of Accidents) say that the majority of these accidents would be prevented if parents remembered the following :

1. To turn pan handles out of reach. No self-respecting toddler can ignore something sticking out just above his head. He has to fetch it down and inspect . . . And that's how he gets three pints of boiling water over him.
2. Never to pass hot drinks over his head. It's not very likely you'll spill any, but why take the risk at all?
3. To keep teapots, kettles and hot-water jugs away from the edge of counters or tables, and to tuck up the tempting overhang of a tablecloth.
4. To keep an eye on the leads of electric kettles and coffee-pots. There's not much point in having the boiling water safely out of reach, if a few good pulls on the attached 'rope' will bring down the kettle or whatever, just the same.
5. To bar Baby from the kitchen when you're sloshing about with buckets of hot water, or transferring food from oven to plates. It's worth putting up with his temporary protest.

6. To teach him by example the rule 'cold before hot' for washing and bathing.

This older baby also is in danger from falls; he still needs to be strapped into his pram or push-chair, and his high-chair. But the worse trouble comes from stairs and windows. Even if he can't reach up to the windows, bear in mind he can drag a chair across and stand on that. So play safe. Use bars or controlled catches. And fix a stair-gate across a flight which he may one day, without anywhere near the necessary skill, decide to climb up or down.

Let's spend a moment on serious injuries. (I'll deal with the small everyday cuts, bruises and stings in the next age-group, where they crop up more frequently.) If your eighteen-month-old has a bad fall—down the cellar steps, for instance—your first impulse will probably be to pick him up and cuddle him. Don't—he may have broken something, in which case he should not be moved until the FRACTURE has been strapped up. Comfort him, of course, in whatever way you know from experience will best reassure him; and meanwhile check for a fracture, probably a greenstick one. (Young children's bones tend to break in the same way as young green twigs—on the outside, with the inside remaining firm.)

If it's a limb that's hurt, get him to try and move it. If he can't do so, then I'm afraid it probably is a fracture. A swelling round the painful area is another give-away, or if the limb appears slightly deformed. Treatment: unless you are miles from the nearest ambulance station—in which case learn in advance about bandaging fractures—I'd advise you to do nothing except dash to a telephone and dial 999. That done, return to keep your small patient company until the experts arrive. Make him comfortable—a cushion under his head, say, and maintain his body temperature. The Red Cross use that phrase because, they say, people are aware they must 'keep the patient warm' and frequently insist on bundling blankets over a fellow too hurt to protest on a boiling hot day! He needs a blanket or coat over him only if he's cold from shock or the weather happens to be cold.

If your toddler appears to have no breakages (I say 'appears' because it is possible that he may complain of pain a day or two later and an X-ray will reveal a crack), then attend to any minor wound. FIRST WASH YOUR HANDS THOROUGHLY. Then with a swab of sterile cotton wool dipped in warm soapy water, remove any loose foreign matter (glass, metal, gravel, etc.) from the wound's surface, but don't go pulling at anything that's embedded. That's a job for the doctor. Gravel out of the way, gently clean the wound with more cotton wool, taking care not to disturb any blood clots. Finally bandage with a prepared sterile dressing. If the bleeding is severe and the blood seeps through the dressing, put another one on top. And in cases where no fracture is suspected, raise the injured part. Then call the doctor or an ambulance. Only an expert can say whether stitches or an anti-tetanus jab are necessary.

I should warn you that in the event of a serious accident, you may find your child UNCONSCIOUS. Don't panic; he'll come round. But call for medical help, as all cases of concussion should be seen by a doctor. And don't assume because he's sitting up crying when you reach him (your toddler, not your overworked G.P.), he didn't lose consciousness at all. He could have done, during that moment it took you to run from the kitchen to the garden. Check if he's dozy. If he can't remember actually colliding with the tree, only running towards it, then he's concussed. And even if he passes your cross-questioning, watch out for mysterious headaches over the next few days.

In conclusion, may I say *never* give a person who has been seriously injured a drink, sweet warm milk or anything else. He may need an anaesthetic, and that necessitates an empty stomach for four hours beforehand. The last thing a loving mother wants to do is to delay an urgent operation, or subject her child to that medical horror: the stomach-pump.

The average home is full of POISONS. Not 007 cyanide files, but plain ordinary cleaning materials. For convenience we usually store these under the sink—which is right on your child's level. Put the saucepans down there instead, and move the deadly bleaches and methylated spirit somewhere else.

Make sure insecticides, weed killers, rat poison, etc., in the garage are not just lying about on the floor. They should be on

a sturdy shelf a good five feet up, or better still locked away in a
cupboard. Bribe father to help.

And then there are medicines—and especially sugar-coated
tablets. Please do keep these in a medicine cabinet, and not
knocking around on your bedside-table. Small children spot
fifty mauve 'sweets' and tuck in—heaven knows with what
results, since they were prescribed for an *adult,* to be taken
one at a time.

I appreciate that if your husband's got an odd pint of prim-
rose paint on a fine Sunday morning and offers to 'run over
Jimmy's cot, or the skirting-board, or his toy truck', the last
thing you want to do is deter him! But before handing him
sand-paper, brush and newspaper, do pause to check the paint
or varnish he intends to use is non-toxic. Babies can suffer from
lead-poisoning if it isn't.

A last comment on the subject of poisons: when your child
is playing outside, look out for lethal plants, like deadly night-
shade, toadstools and laburnum. He hasn't yet outgrown the
habit of putting new things in his mouth, and if the wrong
thing goes in and down, he'll know it!

Or he may not. He may have taken sleeping tablets and be
unconscious. At any event call an ambulance. With poisons
that should be your first move and, if you know what your
child's taken, tell the ambulance men. It could save valuable
analysis time when deciding on the antidote. Then hurry back
and by tickling the back of your child's throat or by giving him
salt-water to drink try to make him vomit. If you *can* get that
poison up, you may prevent it reaching the bloodstream and
doing real harm.

The exception to the vomit rule is if he's swallowed something corrosive like bleach or household disinfectant (look for
blistery burns round his mouth). In this case, dilute the poison
left in his stomach by giving him lots of little drinks of milk, or,
failing that, water.

In the last decade a frightening new killer has emerged on our
domestic scene—the plastic bag. The ghastly part about it is
they're so *useful* in the care of toddlers: ideal for transporting
wet nappies, nice for keeping woollies clean, handy for putting his food in. All right, but *never, never let him get hold of*

one. He can suffocate in seconds if he puts one over his head. (See treatment for ASPHYXIA.) Despite their waterproof quality, don't be tempted to use one as an undersheet; even a fragment of polythene or Cellophane can catch in the throat and obstruct the air passages. In fact in the East this was once used as a method of suicide!

For road-safety what your child really needs is a BSI approved car-seat. I know they're pretty expensive but they're the only totally secure method for him to travel in a car. What's more: they're often designed so that they raise their small passenger to window-level and to have a child who enjoys the car, because he can see out, is such a convenience I'd reckon it's worth foregoing a new dress to afford the seat.

2 – 3½ years

I think we should recap here to something we said in our chapter on Physical Development about teaching your young child to cope with his environment—dangers and all. That's why it is much more valuable to show him how to use scissors, knives, hammers, etc. (in safe, simplified versions), in play than to keep these tools for ever out of his sight. Don't forget, too, that often simple curiosity drives under-fives to fetch down the bread-saw and examine it. If they've never so much as been allowed to see one, let alone been told what it's for and warned, 'Bread-saws have to be very sharp so that we can cut bread with them; that's why we're always careful with them . . .' who can guess what they might do to themselves?

However, once again *gradual* introduction is the operative phrase. Even at three-and-a-half there are many tools too dangerous for him to have access to. A sharpened lawn-mower, for instance, should be shut away at all times; so should razor-blades and the carving-knife.

As you are aware, I'm against frustrating children by *forbidding* them to jump or climb. But you can help your child to become proficient in these skills and thus avoid some of those harder falls. Far better for you and he to have a quiet exploratory 'go' on the climbing-frame, than his first experience of this apparatus to be chasing an older child to the top! Minor tumbles can often be avoided just by doing up a shoe-lace or strap. Your child may not be able to deal with a flapping one himself yet but, if instructed, he can approach an adult for assistance.

With all the knocks and cuts and bruises your child is going to receive, I think it might be helpful if I gave you a basic Medicine Chest.

Plain white gauze in $\frac{1}{2}$ yard pkts. Assorted roller bandages Assorted adhesive dressings Adhesive sticking plaster	These are for minor cuts, which should be washed with soap and water before bandaging.
Polythene bowl Sterile cotton wool balls	Apparatus for above.
Assorted sizes of prepared sterile dressings	For bandaging wounds.
Flannel	To be used soaked in cold water on bruises—*before* they come up.
Medicine glass marked in millimetres	Unless you can convert teaspoonfuls in your head, you're going to need one!
Small pkt. of paper tissues	For wiping away mud, etc.
Safety-pins	Sometimes easier than *tying* a bandage.
Scissors	For cutting the bandages.
Antihistamine cream	For treating insect bites and stings. (First remove the sting, if present. In the event of a sting in the mouth—hospital.)

Paracetamol tablets	To use in place of aspirin, which can have dangerous side-effects in young children.
Calomine lotion	For treating sunburn.
Clinical thermometer	For taking temperature.

Beware of electric sockets. Your child is in far greater danger from them now than he was as a baby with tiny poking fingers. It's unlikely, fortunately, that two fingers will be pushed in simultaneously and far enough. Not so the three-year-old playing with his xylophone hammers. Those long sticks can be inserted in those little holes and *pooooph*! Forbid him to touch electric sockets but I wouldn't count absolutely on his unfailing (and this instance it has to be unfailing) obedience. I'd put blind plugs in them when they're not in use, just to be positive.

If he does somehow manage to ELECTROCUTE himself, first break the contact by switching off the current or, if that is not possible, by standing on dry insulating material (rubber, thickly folded newspaper, book, wood) and using some similar insulating material to knock him clear of the contact. Don't rush up and pull him with bare hands. Electrocuting yourself as well won't save him. Once he's freed, administer first aid in order of precedence:

1. Breathing and heart.
2. Burns.
3. Shock.

Talking of first-aid precedents reminds me to say that almost any road accident involving a young child is a job for the experts. Call an ambulance at once, or make sure someone else does. And I do mean *make sure*. The Red Cross tell me that there are often tragic cases of a dozen or so witnesses to an accident, all convinced somebody else has rung 999.

But while you're waiting for the ambulance to arrive, do the following:

H

1. Preserve life.
   As we've said, this means artificial respiration and
   heart compression as necessary.
   Control bleeding, with firm bandages, and by rais-
   ing the injured part, whenever no fracture is sus-
   pected.
2. Prevent the condition becoming worse.
   Cover wound.
   Immobilise fractures.
   (If necessary, direct traffic *around* casualty)
3. Help recovery.
   Comfort and reassure.
   Protect him from cold.
   Stop spectators crowding round.

But talking of accidents is looking on the black side. I hope
sincerely they will be prevented. On the roads, set your two-
year-old a good example. This is far more valuable than a
hundred lectures and warnings. And when you're on a busy
road, you may find walking-reins are more comfortable than
clutching a tiny paw. You should do one or the other. Of
course, if you have a new baby in a pram as well, and something to carry in your left hand, you are excused. Under
these circumstances train your infant to hold on to the pram.

Very few of us are fortunate enough to have a private swimming-pool (and we can take sour grapes comfort from the
thought that those who have need to watch their children like
hawks) but we may well have an ornamental pond or a water-
butt or even an open drain in our garden. Think about some
protection measure *before* an accident arises.

$3\frac{1}{2}$ – 5 years
Drowning is perhaps an even worse hazard for our last age-
group, because they're often a little way away from home.
They play in a field at the back and drift over to the pond
to look for tadpoles—that sort of thing; you read of such
cases every week in the coroner's court. I realise four-year-olds
want to explore beyond the confines of the garden wall; but
never let your child play unsupervised by water : canals, reser-

voirs, rivers. He is not up to the responsibility yet.

The same goes, of course, when those wet patches are iced over. Forget those delicious Victorian Christmas cards of children skating on the frozen village pond. In this country, especially in the South, we have thin ice that cracks under the weight of a child. Treacherously, it sometimes will hold his weight long enough for him to reach the middle.

And even when your child wants to paddle while the whole family is on the river-bank, take a look yourself first. Currents, sudden shiftings, hidden weeds to trip him up—they can all mean death to a four-year-old. And though you're only feet away, bear in mind river-water is cloudy; you may not be able to find him fast enough.

Just two things to say about his bathing at the seaside. Never let him do so in violation of a red warning flag. The official who hung it up doubtless knows more about that beach than you do. And, besides, it is bad for discipline to encourage your child to defy a civic order. The other thing is rubber air-beds. They're fun, and playing boats on them may help your child to conquer any fear of the water. But don't let him lie on one when you're not right next to him. They can drift out to sea amazingly quickly, especially on an outgoing tide.

Finally, if you are boating with a young child, see that he wears a mini life-jacket.

In the event of DROWNING—The Kiss of Life is slightly different for this older child. You seal your lips round his mouth only, and pinch his nostrils shut with the fingers of one hand, making sure you keep his head well back. And although you blow gently, it'll need to be a little stronger than the puff you'd use for a baby. This time the heart massage is done with the 'heel' of your free hand, and the rocks are slower, only a little above one rock per second.

By now he will probably have outgrown his car-seat (if you've no younger child to take it over, I'd advise you to sell it while the second-hand price is still fairly good) and he will need to be strapped into a BSI approved safety harness—preferably at the back. Actually the seat will probably incorporate a harness you can use.

If he has to walk on the road after dark—always, of course,

accompanied, let him wear something white or, better still, a combined fluoresecent/reflective armband. Once he gets the idea, he'll probably be pretty proud of it.

Now is the age to teach him road-sense properly. Kerb-drill, using the crossing correctly, waiting for a motorist to stop before starting off—these are musts. The local branch of The Tufty Club will do this for you through songs, stories, films and, of course, by playing road safety games. It costs a small fee but the children actually enjoy learning, which is very preferable to a chore they have to go through because Mummy insists. Your Road Safety Officer or police station will gladly inform you about your nearest Tufty Club.

In conclusion I should point out that I have only been able to discuss very general safety problems. RoSPA will help you with one peculiar to you. For instance, they issue an excellent pamphlet on the care of children in agricultural areas.

The same applies to the Red Cross: I've covered only basic First Aid. If you want to learn more, and ideally everyone should, contact your local Red Cross Branch (Address and telephone number in your local directory) about enrolling at one of their classes; and buy their First Aid Wall Chart. It could save you hours of wading through the index at the back of this book every time your child meets with a mishap! The Wall Chart (6 new pence) and the Red Cross's own publication, *ABC of First Aid* (17½ new pence), are both obtainable from their Stores & Supply Department, 4 Grosvenor Crescent, London, S.W.1.

CHAPTER FIFTEEN

In the Eyes of the Law

To MAKE this a comprehensive book about your child under five, I am including a chapter on your financial entitlements and how our legal system affects you both. I hope you'll find the following information useful, though I must admit the odd point is there merely because I found it fascinating and thought you might, too. Although where possible I've stuck to our usual format of starting at birth, or even pre-birth, and working upwards, in this chapter it has usually been more logical to deal with all age-groups while discussing one subject.

BENEFITS

Once your doctor confirms the news you've known for several weeks, you become a privileged being. For a short while your husband carries the shopping; he sits you down and brings tea; perhaps he even buys flowers. Then it dawns on him that this pregnancy lark is going on for months yet, and it's back to normal. Take heart. Though personal privileges may stop, official ones come into play.

That cherished Certificate of Pregnancy from your doctor wins you free dental treatment, the abolition of any charge on the various medicines and tablets prescribed for you (you sign the declaration on the back of each prescription), special cheap vitamin pills obtainable from any Local Authority Clinic, and *if you already have two or more children under five*, seven free pints of milk a week (milk-tokens available from the Welfare Foods Service in Blackpool).

And your local Ministry of Social Security shows its pleasure at your condition in hard cash—stuff called Maternity Grant and Maternity Allowance.

Now, if a married woman is employed, she can opt out of National Insurance contributions (except for the Industrial Accident bit) which saves her about 75p a week, but means she is no longer entitled to sickness benefit, etc. Even if she chooses not to pay, she still gets the Maternity Grant of £25 (not taxable). However, she does not get Maternity *Allowance*, which is £5 weekly for eighteen weeks (also not taxable). To receive that, she must pay *full* contributions for the twelve months ending three months before the expected date of birth.

So it pays you to fork out the full rate if you expect to have a baby within two and three-quarter years. You can change your choice at any time, but a change cannot be back-dated. So it's no good waiting till you're pregnant to pay the full rate (so that you can collect that £90 bonus—£5 x 18—at the end of it). They've thought of that one. You have to make the swap at least six months before conception !

Once your baby is born, as long as he makes at least three children under five or you are what your local Social Security Office count as 'a needy family', you can continue to claim cheap milk by filling up the renewal application at the end of your milk-coupon book. And for all mothers, vitamin pills and baby's concentrated orange-juice and his cod-liver oil (or substitute) come at reduced prices from the Clinic. Other blessings are free medical prescriptions, dental care and optical treatment for children.

A father is entitled to 'child relief' for his children, including a stepchild, or adopted child, or any other child in his custody and maintained by him. For 1971–72 your husband is allowed to deduct from his taxable income £155 per child, so each Smith Junior is worth about £60 to an income tax payer and more to a surtax payer. Even if a child is born on the last day of the tax year—i.e. April 5th, Dad collects the full bonanza for that year. Your husband should claim this by writing to the office of the Inspector of Taxes who handles his earnings, quoting the reference number (they have thousands of files !) and giving them your child's date of birth and full names.

Of course, if you live alone, *you* make the claim. Moreover

if the claimant is a widow, widower, single, separated or div-
orced, or who has a wife who is totally incapacitated throughout the year, he or she is entitled to deduct an additional £100
from taxable income.

Finally, there is Family Allowance. This is paid to families
with two or more children under fifteen (nineteen if still at
school, etc.). So soon after the birth of your second child, you
should obtain a claim-form for Family Allowance tokens at
your local Social Security Office. The allowance at present is
90p a week for two children, £1.90 for three children, £2.90
for four children, and so on with an extra £1 for each additional child. So if you hoard up your tokens, it makes a nice
little packet for expensive items like winter clothes. However,
don't save over years to pay for something like university education; Family Allowances have to be cashed in at the Post Office
within six months of falling due!

Now, although Mother draws the Family Allowance in full,
poor old Father has to fork up tax on it. In order that lower-
paid families should achieve a greater benefit from it than
higher earners, it is taxed as earned income in the ordinary
way. So only families who pay *no* income tax keep the whole
of the Allowance. Furthermore, an additional tax adjustment
is made to take away from income tax-payers the whole of the
£26 p.a. increase given in 1968. But don't despair. Only if your
income is over £10,000 p.a. will every penny you get in Family
Allowance tokens be taken away again in tax.

THE BIRTH CERTIFICATE

But long before you get involved in all these financial claims,
you must register your new baby and the local Medical Officer
of Health must be notified of his arrival. Concealment of birth,
even of a stillborn child, is an offence. If you're muttering
that none of your friends informed the Medical Officer of
Health about their babies, you're probably right. In point of
fact the midwife or doctor in charge of the confinement sees to
this for you.

Moreover, if your baby is born in hospital or a large maternity home, you may well find that the Registrar visits you, which
is very convenient. But if this doesn't happen or if you have the

baby at home, within forty-two days (twenty-one in Scotland)
you or your husband must beetle off to the Register Office of
the district where Junior was born, armed with facts like your
baby's chosen Christian names, and their spellings, the full
names of both parents and grandfathers, the father's occupation and, most important, the date of birth.

One young mother I've heard of spent all the Thursday afternoon and evening in labour and delivered her baby daughter
at half-past twelve, after which she went to sleep for the night.
She blithely informed the Registrar her child was born on
Thursday, and he duly noted down '*11th September*'. Ten
minutes later, she was back to apologise and alter that to the
'*12th*'! Moral: get it sorted out before officialdom confuses you.

In return for this information you will be sent an abbrevi-
ated Birth Certificate (the full version can be purchased for
50p) which you should put away in a safe place, not leave
around on the sideboard with the birth cards and the bootees.
You're going to need to show that Certificate to dozens of
official people in the future.

It may interest you to hear that although this babe-in-arms
is powerless to prevent you calling him Nijinsky—because you
won a lot of money on that horse—he can, when he reaches
maturity, call himself by any forenames of his choice. He
simply introduces himself as 'Sam' and, since we don't usually
ask friends to produce Birth Certificates, nobody will learn
he's really a Nijinsky. That's perfectly legal. If he feels strongly
enough about it, he can even add 'Sam' to his name by deed
poll; but regrettably nothing can strike 'Nijinsky' from the
Certificate. As for his surname—if his father's a Mr Smith,
he becomes a Master Smith; but again on maturity he can call
himself by any other name, or actually *replace* his surname by
deed poll.

If his mother remarries, she is not entitled to change his
surname along with her own. Master Smith remains 'Master
Smith, son of Mrs Brown and stepson of Mr Brown' until he
thinks differently. The trouble is: outsiders tend to assume that
the little boy living with Mr and Mrs Brown is Master Brown
and so, just by usage, he may very well get called 'Brown'
instead of 'Smith'.

If a child is adopted, however, his new parents can change his surname to theirs and give him other forenames. I imagine they would take advantage of this with a new baby dubbed Nijinsky, but not an older child who already knew his name. I'm sure no caring prospective parents would want to confuse, one might almost say dispossess, a three-year-old by telling him he was no longer 'Robbie'.

ADOPTION, FOSTERING, ETC.

But adoption in this country isn't a free-for-all. It's a carefully vetted business which has to be done through a registered adoption society or a local authority. Experts interview would-be adopters, asking endless questions and making extensive inquiries. Religion, income, attitudes, accommodation—their job is to build up a complete picture of this couple who want to adopt. They visit the home in which a child would be brought up, and they visit again later when the child is there. It may sound a bore; it may look like prying. But it's a safeguard for the child; his welfare is too important to bow before personal privacy.

In fact in all legal wrangles *what is best for the child* is regarded as the paramount consideration. Funnily enough the one exception to this rule is right at the outset, when the wishes of the child's natural mother take precedence even above her child's welfare. However seemingly unsuited to the maternal role, she has the right to his custody. And even if she consents to adoption, she can change her mind right up until the Adoption Order is made.

In any case she cannot give her consent until her child is six weeks old. Sometimes the law isn't such an ass. It knows that many an unmarried girl who at six months pregnant talked glibly of 'giving the kid for adoption' feels very differently after she has held and fed and cared for that baby for some weeks. Once she's experienced motherhood, it's quite an ordeal : realising that shortly she will be permanently deprived of her child and all parental rights and duties will rest with the adopters.

Before any Adoption Order is made, however, there must be a probationary period of at least three months. First of all the proposed adopters are given a medical report on the child, and

they in turn have to sign a certificate to say they fully understand what adoption means. Then the child comes to live with
them 'on trial' for anything up to six months. After that, they
either give written notice that they do not want to go ahead
with the adoption or they apply to the Courts for an Adoption
Order.

The Hearing is in private, and the Court keeps the identities
of natural parents and adopters concealed from each other.
Usually the natural parents do not attend the hearing. What
do the Courts look for? Two spouses ideally. Those adopting
through an Agency are bound to be married couples; in the
same way a Court tends to consider favourably an application
from the natural mother or father of the child together with her
or his spouse.

Although the Courts require special justification before plac-
ing a little girl in the charge of a sole male, other instances of
single relatives getting Adoption Orders are common. As long
as they're over eighteen, grandparents (and they're bound to
be over eighteen!), uncles, aunts, brothers, sisters (whether
half-blood or full) are all listened to sympathetically. Where
there is no blood-relationship, one adopter must be at least
eighteen and the other over twenty-five.

By the way, any payment of money in connection with an
adoption other than reimbursement of expenses is strictly
illegal. No democratic law could allow the buying and selling
of babies.

So after the Hearing, it is hoped that the proposed adopters
go home victorious with an Adoption Order. But if there is any
doubt for some reason, occasionally an Interim Order may
be made instead. It gives them a further temporary period of
being parents of anything up to two years at least. A couple of
months before the end of this agonising time, they apply for
the final determination. The heartbreaking thing is that even at
this late stage adoption can be refused. At least, though, the
Court has some discretion. If it is perfectly satisfied that the
adopters are acceptable parents and that the natural parent
has no desire to have the child herself, it can rule that she is
withholding her consent unreasonably and overrule her in
granting the Order.

If a child is over two, he can be consulted with regard to his adoption. Although his *consent* cannot be given in law at any age, it would be heartless to place him with adoptive parents whom he disliked. The Adoption Act provides that the Court shall not make an Adoption Order without 'giving due consideration to the wishes of the infant, having regard to his age and understanding'.

Thus the Courts would not talk to a two-and-a-half-year-old who couldn't understand their questions, and even a four-year-old's answers would be listened to with caution. They appreciate that young children can momentarily 'love' someone who's just given them a Teddy bear and 'hate' an adult who is genuinely dear to them because he or she has recently reprimanded them.

Incidentally, in the event of the death of the natural parents, the law bows, at least initially, to any private wishes expressed by them as regards guardians for their children, whether or not the Court wholly approves the choice. So if you would prefer your best friends rather than certain relatives to take on your offspring if you depart to the hereafter, you'd better say so in writing or preferably in your will. Courts will not accept evidence from the hereafter.

So having had a child, or adopted one (which in law is virtually the same thing) and survived to tell the tale, one is responsible for him. One may even use reasonable force to protect him. Certainly one must house, maintain and rear one's child. Under the Children and Young Persons Act 1933, the parent who neglects or abandons his child in a way likely to endanger or cause suffering to his health is almost as bad as the one who uses active physical violence.

If a Local Authority sees that a child's welfare demands it, it must receive him into care. This means moving him into one of its own children's homes or boarding him out with foster parents, who incidentally are paid.

If the child has been removed because of temporary sickness or homelessness on the part of his parents, it is hoped that he can be reunited with them shortly. But sometimes this is not possible and he finds himself living for more than a decade with foster parents. As you've doubtless read, the whole law with regard to fostering is under review, owing to some heart-rending cases of natural mothers reclaiming their children from the only 'Mummy' they've ever known.

Yet despite the general, very real affection between children and their foster parents, every Local Authority keeps a close eye on its foster homes, making inspections from time to time and imposing certain conditions, like the number of foster children allowed or some stipulation about accommodation. The Authorities recognise that any child being fostered has suffered one emotional upheaval and must be protected from the risk of another. If they consider the household unsuitable, they can apply to the Juvenile Court, which, if satisfied, will remove the child.

But assuming you and your husband are going to care for your child, both physically and morally, it may interest you to learn that the lion's share of the responsibility and the prerogatives rests with the male lion. Whilst I sincerely hope you're going to bring up your children jointly and make joint decisions about them, if you are in dispute, English law (for centuries, of course, compiled by men) favours the father. He chooses his child's religion; it is his consent which is required for an operation; he must give written agreement for his child's name to be added to the mother's passport; he has the right to the custody of his legitimate child (and a child is legitimate if his natural parents marry *at any time*) over and above the mother. Yes! In practice, though, he seldom gets it with a child under five.

DIVORCE

The subject of custody is most relevant, of course, when the parents split up, and Divorce Court judges take the view that a very young child should remain with his mother. When she is what used to be called 'the guilty party' but a good loving mother none the less, the Court may give her care and control but leave custody—the legal bit—with her ex-husband.

It says a lot for British compromise that whichever parent doesn't gain 'care and control' or custody usually gets 'reasonable access' to visit the children, and on the whole this works, without argument. Only if the parents are too hostile towards each other to cope with such a fluid arrangement will the Court lay down an arrangement like 'every Sunday and six weeks in the summer' . . .

Let's take a look at divorce under the new laws (operative since 1 January, 1971). The fact that a man no longer wishes to live with his wife doesn't let him out of housing and maintaining her and their children. He must provide a roof over their heads, and just because he owns the house doesn't entitle him to turn them out. In fact for some roving husbands it could be grimmer than that. The Court may even rewrite the title deeds, changing the ownership of the property as they see fit.

As far as money's concerned, a deserted wife, whose husband leaves her without a penny, can go to her local magistrate's court (on legal aid if eligible) and ask it to order the husband to pay so much a week. At once. Accordingly, the Bench makes a Maintenance Order of 'such sum as it considers reasonable in all the circumstances'. As you gather, that gives the Court a lot of discretion. They realise that a wife with three children might well need, for example, £16 a week but if the father is earning only £22 after deductions, then it's just not on. They appreciate that he also has rent to pay and food to buy, and if he is living with another woman he may have her children to support in addition; so the wife would be lucky to wind up with £10 a week. It comes to the fact that inevitably *both* parties will have to reduce their standards of living.

Even a wronged wife's standard of living must not be 'significantly higher' than her husband's. The Court does not set out to *punish* him for immorality; immorality may be undesirable, but it is not illegal. A mother whose four or five-year-old is out at school may have her Maintenance Order reduced on the grounds she could add to her own income by working part-time if for instance she used to work before she was married. It seems it just doesn't pay any more to play 'wronged wife' for the rest of one's life, and one certainly can't deny a man his divorce because he'll take it anyway after five years of the marriage irretrievably breaking down.

If one's estranged husband packs his bags in a civilised way, leaving £9 a week for housekeeping and children's clothes and promising to continue meeting the mortgage and the gas bill and the rates, then one will probably wait for the Court to make this a formal Court Order—with a Maintenance Order for the children until they are sixteen and for oneself. There's still one hitch, though. In Scotland, Maintenance Orders are, like income tax, deducted from wages at source; but in England and Wales it's up to the honesty of the husband to pay up regularly. Many a sad wife whose husband started off gallantly has to re-apply to the Court for mounting arrears, and then the Court may order his employer to deduct Maintenance at source—known as an Attachment of Earnings Order.

CIVIL AND CRIMINAL ACTION

A one-year-old may bring a legal action. The case is brought on his behalf by his 'next friend', generally speaking his father or mother. If an action is brought *against* him, then he defends through his 'guardian ad litem'—again Father or Mother.

Since any child under ten years is presumed to be too young to be capable of forming the necessary intent to commit a crime, your small son or daughter cannot be held guilty of a criminal offence. You and I may know differently, but that's the law and be thankful for it.

As for civil wrongs, an infant is responsible for his misdeeds only if he is of such an age that he can distinguish between right and wrong. The four-year-old who maliciously throws bricks through your next-door-neighbour's window is considered not to know the difference. Still, I don't think we'll tell him that—bad for discipline. However, sometimes you, as his parents, can be held responsible. If, for example, you gave him a dangerous article like a shotgun to play with, and he shot someone in the leg with it, then you might have to answer for that injury, on the grounds that you had not exercised sufficient control over the gun or hadn't supervised your child properly.

In all civil proceedings the 'next friend' or 'guardian ad litem' as the case may be, can act only if he or she is not connected with the case adversely to the interests of the infant. For instance, if a child was entitled to claim against his father for injuries resulting from an accident he caused, then the child would have to sue through his mother. Whenever damages in an action are awarded to a child, they are paid into Court, and the Court then watches over the money and must approve its investment. At any event, the money is *not* paid out of Court until the child attains majority (eighteen). This is to prevent greedy parents saying that little Jimmy's 'bad foot money' should buy them a colour television, leaving him bereft. After all, a four-year-old doesn't understand about his financial rights in a Trust the way he does about 5p pieces in his money-box! He knows when you've scrounged one of those for the gas meter.

Incidentally, if a Settlement is reached by negotiation (instead of a Court decision), then a Court may still be asked to approve the Settlement, to make sure it is a fair one. But this is not compulsory.

PROPERTY

A child can acquire property by gift or inheritance. In the case of land it must be put into the name of trustees, and this is frequently also done in the case of other property, such as investments—especially if the person giving it wishes to make conditions, for example that the property is to go to Cousin Willie if the original infant does not reach a certain age. Except where the will or deed of gift states otherwise, the trustees may pay the whole or part of the income to the child's parent or guardian for his maintenance, education or benefit. The remaining income must be invested and accumulated at compound interest until the child becomes eighteen. In some cases, where the child needs it, some of the capital also can be spent on him.

A father may be a trustee, but he does not have any rights over his child's property. He holds it only as an agent would. Poor old Dad. If he buys property in his child's name, he is presumed to have made a gift to the child.

This is also so, morally if not legally, with Premium Bonds. You know—parents buy their child one each year on birthdays to build up a nest-egg for him. And then one May morning Ernie coughs up £50,000 for that child! Well, the prize is *his*, even though the parents' money bought the Bond origin-

ally. Granted, the Post Office pay up to the parents, but it is to
be hoped that they will regard themselves as *trustees*, not
owners, of the win and spend or invest the money to their
child's advantage.

A child can have a current bank account but the bank will
not allow him to overdraw it because, if he did, the bank
could not recover the debt in law. An infant in our age-group
may also have a bank deposit account. However, deposits
in this, the National Savings Bank and the Trustee Savings
Bank have to be made through another person (a two-year-
old can't sign his name) and cannot be withdrawn unless it is
shown that the amount is needed again for the infant's maintenance or benefit. So as a general rule : what goes in, stays in.

Unless a company's Articles of Association expressedly pro-
hibit it or some wary company secretary refuses to register him,
there is nothing to stop an under-five owning shares. Or rather,
I suppose, having shares bought for him. Once he is the registered shareholder, the dividends would be his, paid to him by
cheque or direct into that bank account he possesses. (If, by the
way, you're thinking by now that your own child is somewhat
financially deprived, let me reassure you that none of *my* children had the odd bit of diamond stock, nor even—for shame—
his own bank account!) Anyway, to carry it one further :
technically this loaded eighteen-month-old could toddle into
the Annual General Meeting clutching two plastic bricks and
a clean nappy, and raise his hand in favour of voting the
directors off the Board !

At the end of the financial year, all Junior's unearned income will have to be declared for tax purposes. But, of course,
there is no interest (and therefore no tax) on Premium Bonds;
the appreciation on National Savings Certificates is tax-free,
and anyone can hold up to £600 in the National Savings
Bank before paying tax on the interest.

And if your child is so wealthy he has the maximum tax-
free holding in all these and he has to fork out $38\frac{3}{4}\%$ tax on
things like share dividends, do you think I'm going to *sympathise*?

As for *earned* income (and I'm going to deal with Employment of Children at the end of this chapter), a child, like any-

one else, is allowed to earn £418 p.a. before paying any income tax.

BABY-MINDERS

I am sure you will remember those ghastly exposés on baby-minding of a few years back. Well, in 1968 an Act was passed which stated that anyone wishing to mind one or more children (who are not relatives) under school age, for reward, for two hours or more daily must be registered with their Local Authority.

If you want to be a registered child-minder, it won't cost you anything to be accepted; but it will submit you to certain, very reasonable conditions. First of all you and anyone over sixteen who lives in your house or is going to assist you in this venture must be in good physical and mental health and must have had a recent chest X-ray confirming freedom from tuberculosis. And none of you can have been convicted of any offence in connection with children or have had a child removed from your care by Court Order. I should think not indeed!

Once you've signed the declaration to say that so far you're in the clear, an officer from the Public Health Department will visit your home to make an inspection. He or she will want to know that the place is hygienic, the sanitary facilities are adequate and that there is room and apparatus for play. He will also check up on safety hazards and fire risk. Finally you will be told how many (if any) infants you may mind. Defy that decision at your peril: for local council officers have a duty to satisfy themselves that the children in your care are making satisfactory progress, and have the right to make further visits at any time. So if they say 'three children' and you take on six, you're likely to be found out!

Having passed the inspection, you're all set to go into business. There may, however, be certain additional local requirements. For instance, one London Borough I know of also ask baby-minders to keep a list with the name and address of each child, their dates of birth, the mothers' places of employment and the telephone numbers, and the names and addresses of the children's G.P.s. Apparently they'd had cases of little Doris being taken queer and the baby-minder having no idea who

242   THE NEW CHILDHOOD

Doris's *mother* was, let alone her doctor! The baby-minder reported that Doris's mother was a dark-haired lady who lived somewhere nearby and dropped off the little girl each morning at a quarter-to-nine! Obviously some more definite records needed to be kept.

(Incidentally, if you are taking up baby-minding, you may like to contact your council about voluntary training schemes and about the loan of play equipment.)

I'm sure no fair-minded person would quarrel with the above legislation. It is designed wholly to protect your child, who is, after all, too young to protect himself. Basically, the law recognises that your child is an individual in his own right but it is nevertheless there to protect his interests and safeguard his position, as he is too young to look out for himself. He is protected against anything, whether it be a contract or an evil guardian or anything else, which would be to his disadvantage.

PROTECTION

Although there is no law to prevent a one-year-old sitting through a nude show on the stage, he is forbidden to enter a cinema showing a film with an AA or X certificate. Personally I don't relish the idea of any child under three being taken to the pictures, since his comprehension wouldn't stretch to even Walt Disney (compare how much simpler tots' television is) and he'd grow very bored with sitting still for a couple of hours. Moreover, little dramas, like the sight of a witch, can work on the imagination of a very young child and terrify him out of his wits.

But if you insist, the law won't stop you. Before your child is one, you can take him into anything, because the official view is he's a babe-in-arms and therefore incorruptible. I quarrel with that. As I said in 'A Member Of The Family', even a very new baby can be subconsciously aware of a sexual or violent atmosphere, which is bad for him. When discussing phobias, we mentioned his fear of sudden loud noises. So when the rest of the audience cheers as the good cowboys gun down the baddies, your baby is much more likely to burst into tears. And then what are you going to do? You can't keep him there bawling and disturbing everyone else, and you don't want to take him out because you'll miss the rest of the film yourself. Far, far better to leave him at home with the sitter; the air's fresher for him, too.

Incidentally, where the majority of a theatre or cinema audience is children, there must be sufficient adults to supervise them. In the case of a fire, for instance, it would require more than a couple of usherettes to herd several hundred four-year-olds safely out of the emergency exits.

On the killer subject of fire in connection with young children, the law has tried to make some rules. Reformers might well like to go the whole way and make it an offence to leave a child alone in a room with a fire that's alight, but they know any such law would be unenforceable. How would the police know that child was with the oil stove playing in the living-room, while Mother was outside gardening? They would know only if that child was killed or seriously injured and that led them to make investigations. So the law has compromised. If a young child is killed or seriously injured by a fire or other heating appliance due to his parent (or person over sixteen to whom the parent has temporarily delegated his care) not taking reasonable precautions for his safety, then that adult is answerable in criminal law. In any event, it is against the law to sell an unguarded fire.

It is an offence to allow any kind of literature which could corrupt Junior (with regard to our age-group it would have to be in picture-form) to fall into his hands.

And it is also an offence to give any child under five intoxicating liquor, unless prescribed by a doctor or otherwise justified. I suspect the law is really after the woman who gives her baby gin each evening to keep him quiet, rather than the Daddy who lets his small son taste his beer or the mother who lets her baby daughter suck her finger doused in christening champagne. Still, technically such goings-on are breaking the law. Doubtless you are already aware that you cannot take your child into a pub during opening hours—a law perpetuated by fathers, I suspect, who use the pub as a refuge from their families! And it is also an offence to sell alcohol to children.

Ah yes, and if you should wish to tattoo 'KISS ME QUICK' across your little lad's chest, you'll have to find a doctor who sympathises with such a curious desire! Since 1969, tattooing (and this is defined as 'the insertion into the skin of any colouring material designed to leave a permanent mark') a minor can be performed only by a qualified doctor. The mind boggles at the thought of what may have gone on prior to 1969 . . .

EMPLOYMENT

After the Dickensian horrors of child labour, no wonder we have stringent statutes that forbid the employment of young children, paid or unpaid. However, recently there has been a vast increase in the need for children in entertainment and advertising. Though men may drool over bikini-clad birds, any copywriter worth his expense-account will tell you that the way to hook a woman is by showing her children under five years of age.

Hence, 2,000 kids regularly—and many thousands more on a casual basis—are permitted to take part in films and plays, to pose for baby-food ads for television, etc., providing the persons responsible for the performance have the signed support of the parents on a special form, and then obtain a licence from the Local Authority consenting to the participation of the children. That way the Authority can assure itself that certain conditions are being observed:

1. That the part cannot be taken *except* by a child of about this age.
2. That the child's health and education will not suffer, and that he won't be endangering life or limb.
3. That during the previous twelve months, he hasn't taken part in other performances on more than thirty-nine days—49 under special circumstances.
4. That the applicant will keep records (for example, of attendances, etc).
5. That both licence applicant and parents understand that the money earned belongs to the child. The Local Authority can insist that the sum be paid into the County Court (Sheriff's Court in Scotland) and ad-

ministered for the child, or alternatively dealt with in a way approved by the Authority.

6. That the child won't work more than the allowed number of hours.

Those hours for our age-group are as follows:

A. A child shall be present at the studio no more than five hours a day (three hours for two-year-olds and under).

b. He shall not *work* for more than two hours per day (one hour for two-year-olds and under).

c. He must not work for more than thirty minutes continuously without a rest (twenty minutes for two-year-olds and under).

d. He shall not work before 9.30 a.m. and after 4.30 p.m.

However, no licence is required where the performance is for charity or under an arrangement with the school (presumably because the above protection can then be taken for granted); or if a child has not performed on more than three days in the preceding six months. So all but the really professional mini entertainers are employed without licences. The number of hours they are permitted to work still stand; but generally they look to their mothers and the studios for protection rather than the law. And that's far from satisfactory. The studio's prime interest is in getting the job done, and all too often it is the mothers who are stage-struck.

Heartlessly, they drag their good-looking offspring from audition to audition, and when, or if, that's successful, from shooting to shooting . . . often waiting hours with them in draughty dressing-rooms. Their reward: reflected glory when they see little Johnnie on TV or in a magazine, his reward: about £10 less heavy expenses per *working* day.

Some producers are absolutely marvellous with young children; but to lots of others the children are an enigma, who, compared with adult actors, are slow to learn lines and gestures and who do not appreciate the essentials of facing the camera and grinning at the product. Producers have a schedule to meet and dislike wasting time while scores of their cast trot off to the lavatory. They explain to a three-year-old that this—some beautiful remote model totally unused to children—is Mummy, and are perplexed when the little girl or boy bursts into tears and clings to his or her real mother.

Do I need to spell it out any more? I strongly believe that encouraging, virtually insisting, a child makes an exhibition of himself regularly is almost bound to turn him out precocious and very conscious of himself. But worse than that is the fact it's putting emphasis on such superficial qualities, like cuteness instead of on character. Also pity the child for the psychological effect on him of having a mother who needs him to SUCCEED as a star; it's several degrees worse than the mother who wants her child to walk before the small fellow next door. And make no mistake: however it winds up, originally it was the *mother* who fancied this 'career'. After all, two-year-olds don't know about modelling. The whole business is comparable with the father who puts his eighteen-year-old son into medicine because that's the profession he secretly hankers after himself.

I have only scratched the surface of the law with regard to your child under five. If you have a legal problem in this context and you don't have a solicitor to consult, contact your local Citizens Advice Bureau, who will give detailed advice.

CHAPTER SIXTEEN

Off to School

As YOUR child reaches the end of the age-span of this book—in other words five—he will start proper school. Emotionally, socially and educationally, this would be a vast step away from being at home all day with you, playing with whichever toy suits his fancy at any particular moment. So, true to my gradient scale principle, I believe your child should first take the intermediary step of attending nursery school or Playgroup.

Already, through being left with baby-sitters, he has learned to get along happily without you for brief periods; pre-school education will now afford him the opportunity of coping without you on a regular basis—anything from a couple of mornings a week to five full schooldays. So when the inevitable 9 o'clock till 3.15 parting arrives, it won't be a painful wrench.

At proper school, too, your child will be expected to be respectful to, but certainly not terrified of, a teacher and to work in a class full of other children. That's a bit different from what we discussed in 'Your Child and Other Animals'—about being polite to the odd friend who drops in for a cup of tea or playing contentedly for an hour with the little girl next door. Another reason why pre-school education is useful.

Finally it is invaluable in teaching your child *how to learn*. In a moment I shall mention what goes on at nursery school and Playgroup and you will see that, although there is no formal teaching (alphabet, counting, reading, etc.), his mind is stimulated in a way that encourages him to want to find out. At proper school the pupil who wants to know is the pupil who gets on.

Doubtless the Ministry of Education would be the first to agree with all these sound reasons for Britain's under-fives attending nursery school; but it's a matter of expenditure. Generally speaking, universities, technical colleges, secondary and primary schools have had to take precedent over nursery schools. Nevertheless, there are some (though not nearly enough) State nursery schools in existence, and during the Sixties many primary schools opened up nursery classes.

Both nursery schools and nursery classes are quite distinct from *Day nurseries*—which are in effect State baby-minders. Day nurseries grew up to help mothers, mainly mothers who for one reason and another *had* to go out to work, by taking care of their under-fives (very often babies and toddlers) during the day. State nursery schools, on the other hand, were established for the benefit of the *children*, regardless of the needs of the parents. Even so, the pupils have to be selected on an evaluation of need : for there are always more applicants than places. Thus it might be decided that a four-year-old who suffered from a speech deficiency needed the constant chatter of children at nursery school more than another child without that handicap.

There are also *private* nursery schools, many of which are run by excellent qualified teachers who use various different approaches to pre-school education. For instance, the permissive Froebel approach or the much more disciplined approach of the Montessori school. 'Disciplined' does not mean that the children sit at tiny desks facing the blackboard on which the teacher does her 'chalk and talk' routine. But the exponents of the Montessori system will I am sure agree that their handling of education follows a more formal pattern.

Beware the few lingering Miss So-and-so's kindergartens round the corner. Some of them may be good, but some cling to rigid lessons, which are valueless and unsuitable for our age-group.

Fees vary from £2 to £4 per week and they have whole-day and half-day arrangements and orange-juice and dinner may be included for your money.

So the first thing to do is contact your Health Visitor and ask whether there is a nursery school near you. And 'near', in our age-group, is an operative word. A couple of miles' bus journey away is probably no good. Your three-year-old cannot travel on his own and, unless you are fortunate enough to have a car, taking him there every morning and collecting him at 12.15 is going to prove an awful bind.

But even if you find a nearby nursery school, State or private, you will be lucky if your child is admitted, owing to the shortage of places . . . which is why the 'amateur' version of nursery school has grown up—Playgroup. However, although Playgroup leaders are not qualified teachers as such, the Playgroups Association run comprehensive courses to train them: so you need have no fear that your child will be in the hands of someone who hasn't a clue what she's doing.

And what are they doing in a Playgroup? I can do no better than to quote from the Playgroups Association's own pamphlet:

PLAYMATES—A child enjoys himself within the framework of a group. He learns to respect other people and to feel secure with his contemporaries and with adults even when his parents are not there.

PLAYTHINGS—Indoors and out: study, carefully selected educational play equipment and material for creative activities extend a child's abilities. From his growing ability springs confidence, pleasure and increased interest in the world around.

PLAYSPACE—Room to run, dance, climb and use all his faculties and developing muscles in every possible way.

PLAYTIME—Time to concentrate, to pursue an idea, whether building a rocket or digging a hole. Time to finish the job before he must clear it away.

It would be unfair to say that *all* Playgroups are equally well-equipped. Obviously those run in private houses for perhaps only half a dozen children cannot be expected to be as enterprising as an old-established one for thirty children in a large hall with a big field at the back. But somebody's private house (yours if nobody else has volunteered) is far better than nothing.

Throughout this book I have spoken of your child's need for companionship, increasingly companionship from his contemporaries. And I have spoken of his need for a 'child-orientated environment'—somewhere where everything is there for the child's purpose : where the only 'nos' are those that are strictly anti-social, like hitting your 'friend' over the head.

So when is your child ready for nursery school or Playgroup? Well, *they* won't take *him* before he's two and out of nappies. That's reasonable. Remember, they are not a nursery; those teachers and leaders are there to stimulate his development, not to waste their talents changing wet nappies all day long. But in point of fact many will not take entrants until three. Very rightly, they argue that it is better to fill their limited places with children between three and five, who dearly *need* pre-school education, than with younger children for whom it would be enjoyable.

Now whilst I believe that *all* children should be encouraged and given opportunity to play with their contemporaries, I am not going to be so foolish as to state that each one is ready at two-and-a-half or three or three-and-a-half to leave his mother regularly and go off to Playgroup or nursery school for three hours each morning. In this, as in everything, your child is an individual. Some children, despite having gradually been weaned away from you with sitters, are not ready for this break as early as others. Some, like my son, are ready to go off at fourteen months!

When he was this age, Merle went to nursery school and Tina to proper school, and both sisters obviously looked forward to rushing off to this thing called 'school'. His great cry of frustration every morning as he sat in his high-chair finishing his toast and watching them gaily leaving was: 'Chool!' I told him that fourteen months was too young for school; but it still took me most of the rest of the morning to get him to play contentedly at home.

Then when he was almost sixteen months old I took the bull by the horns and went along to the nursery school where his sister was going, and I told the teacher my problem. 'I have a sixteen-month-old child who wants to come to nursery school; what shall I do?'

And she said: 'Oh dear . . . well, you know I can't take him.' But I still stood there, and she thought about it and, being a very understanding person who knew about children, she said: 'Tell me: can he eat entirely independently?'

And I said: 'Almost.'

She said: 'Can he walk entirely on his own?'

'Nearly.'

'Good. When he can eat by himself, when he can walk, and when he's potty-trained, bring him to me—and, if necessary, we'll hide him from the inspectors!'

So when Nicholas was eighteen months old he went to nursery school every day, and there was once a situation where he *was* hidden from the inspectors—in the upstairs lavatory actually! He attended fulltime, from the first day onwards, because he was so happy there he refused to come home at lunchtime.

But he was exceptional, and so was that nursery school teacher. As a general rule, I would say that eighteen months is the time to find out what is available for your child in your area, and at what age they will admit him. But don't take anyone else's word for whether your local nursery class, private nursery school or Playgroup is good or bad. Read up about the various approaches to nursery education and buy Brenda Crowe's book *Playgroup Activities* (Price 25p) from Pre-school Playgroups Association, 87a, Borough High Street, London, S.E.1. Then GO AND SEE FOR YOURSELF before you make your decision.

Now, while your child is attending pre-school education, you have to think about the future.

PRIMARY SCHOOL

It is advisable to investigate local primary schools long before your child is five. Many have lists for places on which they take the names of four-year-olds. If you want to send your child to a church school or a private fee-paying school, the lists open earlier: sometimes when the children are two.

The person to inform you of all the schools available to you is your Local Authority Education Officer. He can tell you about your rights and duties as a parent of a school-age child, and answer specific questions about things like the religious instruction your child will receive or the bus-pass he may be entitled to.

Take time over selecting your primary school. And don't be afraid to phone for an appointment to meet the head-teacher, so that you can ask him about his school. It is our job as parents not only to choose wisely, so that the child's school will be the right one for him, but also to prepare him emotionally so that he's ready to get the best out of school.

If he has gone to nursery school or nursery class fulltime before this moment, the transition will be looked forward to eagerly. After all, going to 'proper school' is promotion. Mother, too, will be used to being parted from him for regular long periods each day. But if he has only had part-time pre-school education, he is bound to feel strange, tired and a little overwhelmed at first. Don't be alarmed by this or by a temporary change in his behaviour at home. Accept this with understanding and patience; it should soon pass.

All mothers feel nostalgic that their 'baby' has grown up; that's natural. The point is not to be *sad*. Be proud instead—your child has taken his first big step on the road to maturity.

Index

Books for parents in Tandem editions

The Womanly Art of Breastfeeding 25p
For every mother who has ever wondered about the
relative advantages of breastfeeding and bottle-feeding

Infant Care 25p
Everything you should know about caring for your baby
from birth to one year old

A Time for Joy Martha Blount 25p
Sound practical advice on every aspect of childhood, with
chapters devoted to the gifted child, the late developer,
the handicapped or disabled child

Points for Parents Elizabeth Longford 30p
Answers to most family problems, inspired by other
parents' letters to the author

Teaching an Infant to Swim Virginia Hunt Newman (Illus.) 25p
'It is never too soon to teach a child water-safety'

Books for the family in Tandem editions

By Spike Milligan
The Little Pot-Boiler 25p
A Book of Bits or a Bit of a Book 25p
A Dustbin of Milligan 25p
The Bedside Milligan 25p

By Jonathan Always
More Puzzles to Puzzle You 20p
What! More Puzzles? 25p
Puzzles? You're Joking! 25p
Puzzles for Puzzlers 25p

Sullivan's Second Book of Crossword Puzzles 20p
Sullivan's Third Book of Crossword Puzzles 20p